Board Review

HISTOLOGY

BOARD REVIEW SERIES

HISTOLOGY

LESLIE P. GARTNER, Ph.D.
Associate Professor of Anatomy
University of Maryland
Dental School
Baltimore, Maryland

JAMES L. HIATT, Ph.D.
Associate Professor of Anatomy
University of Maryland
Dental School
Baltimore, Maryland

JUDY M. STRUM, Ph.D.
Professor of Anatomy
University of Maryland
School of Medicine
Baltimore, Maryland

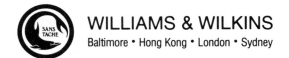

WILLIAMS & WILKINS
Baltimore • Hong Kong • London • Sydney

Editor: Kim Kist
Associate Editor: Victoria M. Vaughn
Copy Editor: Elizabeth M. Cowley
Design: Norman Och
Illustration Planning: Lorraine Wrzosek
Production: Raymond E. Reter

Copyright © 1988
Williams & Wilkins
428 East Preston Street
Baltimore, MD 21202, USA

Printed in the United States of America

Library of Congress Cataloging in Publication Data

Gartner, Leslie P., 1943–
    Histology / Leslie P. Gartner, James L. Hiatt, Judy M. Strum.
      p. cm. — (Board review series)
    Includes index.
    ISBN 0-683-03434-0
    1. Histology.   I. Hiatt, James L., 1934–   II. Strum, Judy M.
  (Judy May)   III. Title.   IV. Series.
    [DNLM: 1. Histology. QS 504 G2435h]
  QM551.G37 1988
  611′.018—dc19
  DNLM/DLC
  for Library of Congress   87-31757
                                             CIP

91 92

3   4   5   6   7   8   9   10

PREFACE

The purpose of this book is to help students review the massive amount of material that comprises Histology. Although our intent is to assist those preparing for National Board Examinations, this book is also a valuable tool and study aid to review for class examinations. It is designed in a format that maximizes a student's efforts.

This book is composed of 19 chapters. Each chapter is organized so that the first few paragraphs give a general overview of the material to be covered. Then the subject is divided into several major and minor headings. These subdivisions are clearly indicated, so that readers may skip the areas that are familiar to them. Under each subheading key words (or phrases) and their descriptions, definitions, or explanations are provided. The prime reason for using this format is that it permits one to view the material at a glance, rather than having to spend time ferreting out particular points. The key words are set apart for a second reason, that they might conjure up a sequence of images and factual information in the student's mind, providing instant feedback as to what must be reviewed prior to an examination. In each chapter the functional aspects are treated under a separate heading, which may be studied either with or apart from the descriptive matter. The chapters are enhanced with excellent illustrations that facilitate the review of the material. Each chapter concludes with a series of about 15 questions (in the style of National Board questions), followed by annotated answers.

We would like to thank our many friends at Williams & Wilkins, including Norman Och for excellence of design; our copy editor Elizabeth M. Cowley; our editors Vicky Vaughn and Kim Kist; Ray Reter our production editor; Pamela Caras for her constant efforts in promoting our endeavors; John Gardner, Editor-in-Chief and Vice President, for asking us to write this book; and finally Sarah Finnegan, President, for her continued support. A special thanks to our respective families for the support they have always given in these undertakings.

We hope that this review book will be effective in preparing students for the various examinations "that flesh is heir to." Although we have endeavored to be accurate and complete, we realize that shortcomings, errors, and omissions may occur in an undertaking of this type. Therefore, we welcome criticisms, suggestions, and comments that will assist us in improving it.

Baltimore

Leslie P. Gartner
James L. Hiatt
Judy M. Strum

CONTENTS

1
The Cell

The Cell

—is the smallest unit of living matter capable of independent existence.
—contains two major compartments: nucleus and cytoplasm.
—nucleus contains chromatin, consisting of genetic material.
—cytoplasm contains organelles (metabolically active units of living matter), inclusions (inert accumulations of material), and the cytoskeleton.

Nucleus

Characteristics
—contains the genetic apparatus encoded in the DNA of chromosomes.
—directs protein synthesis in the cytoplasm via macromolecules of ribosomal RNA (rRNA), messenger RNA (mRNA), and transfer RNA (tRNA).
—displays euchromatin: lightly stained, dispersed chromatin in the process of being transcribed.
—displays heterochromatin: densely stained, condensed chromatin, not currently being transcribed.

Chromosome Organization
—is complex, consisting of multiple coils and supercoils.
—coils are composed of nucleosome cores of histones with a DNA double helix wrapped around them.

Nuclear Envelope
—consists of two parallel membranes separated from each other by a narrow perinuclear space.
—the inner and outer nuclear membranes are continuous with one another around the nuclear pores, which interrupt the double membrane of the envelope.

Outer Nuclear Membrane
—has ribosomes attached and is continuous with the endoplasmic reticulum.

Inner Nuclear Membrane
—contains a thin meshwork of interwoven intermediate filaments, called the fibrous lamina (nuclear lamina).
—fibrous nuclear lamina serves as an anchoring site for interphase chromosomes.

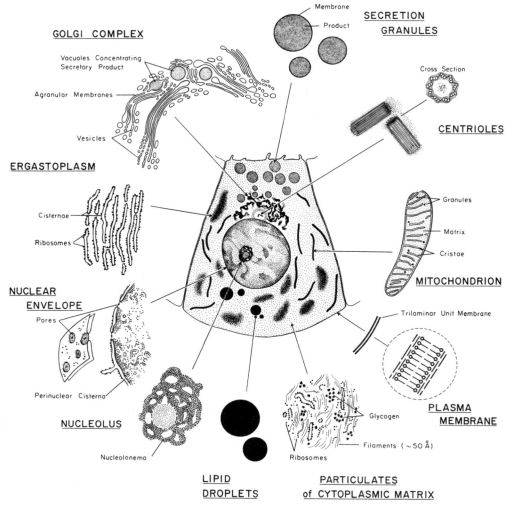

Figure 1.1. Drawing of the fine structure of the cell, its organelles, and inclusions. (From Fawcett DW: *Bloom and Fawcett's Textbook of Histology*, ed 11. Philadelphia, WB Saunders, 1986.)

Nuclear Pore

—consists of a membrane-bounded, octagonal channel between the nucleus and the cytoplasm.

—the outer and inner nuclear membranes are continuous around each pore.

—is associated with the "nuclear pore complex," consisting of several nonmembranous structures:

—a centrally located electron-dense granule (plug).

—eight large protein granules arranged in an octagonal pattern that define the inner and outer rim of each pore.

—eight radially arranged spokes extending from the eight granules into the center of the pore.

—provides communication between the nucleus and the cytoplasm.

—varies in number and distribution, depending on cell type and stage of differentiation.

Nucleolus

—a well-defined nuclear inclusion (sometimes more than one) observed in cells that are actively synthesizing protein.

—electron micrographs reveal three typical regions:

  —fibrillar component of 5 nm diameter fibrils that represent early stages in the formation of rRNA precursors;

  —granular component of 15 nm particles that represent later stages in the formation of rRNA precursors;

  —nucleolar-associated chromatin, consisting of DNA from the nucleolar organizer region of chromosome.

—involved in synthesis of rRNA and its packaging into precursors of ribosomes.

Cytoplasm

Organelles

Plasma Membrane (plasmalemma, cell membrane)

—surrounds cell and forms boundary between it and the outside world.

—consists of a phospholipid bilayer within which integral proteins are distributed.

—the hydrophilic ends of the phospholipids face outward; their hydrophobic chains project inward.

—freeze-fracture preparations (from enzymatically active cells) reveal more protein particles on the P face than on the E face.

—proteins occupy different positions within the bilayer:

  —some are fixed in the membrane by certain cytoskeletal components.

  —others move laterally within the plane of the membrane.

Glycocalyx (surface coat)

—exists on the external surface of the plasma membrane.

—formed primarily by polysaccharide components of integral membrane glycoproteins and glycolipids.

—imparts a negative charge to the cell surface.

—plays a role in immunological specificity.

—contains blood group antigens, has receptor sites, and acts as a protective mechanical barrier.

—in cells of the small intestine contains enzymes that hydrolyze disaccharides and polypeptides, thus functioning in digestion.

Ribosomes

—particles measuring 12×25 nm, which consist of a large and a small subunit.

—composed of rRNA and a number of proteins.

—often cluster together in groups along a strand of mRNA to form polyribosomes (polysomes).

—synthesize protein, after becoming associated with mRNA.

Rough Endoplasmic Reticulum (RER)

—a system of sheets and cavities bounded by membranes whose outer surface is studded with ribosomes.

—has an interior region that is called the cisterna.

—has receptors (specific glycoproteins, called ribophorins) in its membranes to which the large subunit of the ribosome binds, while the mRNA strand occupies a cleft in the small subunit of the ribosome.

—is common in cells synthesizing proteins for export (secretory proteins).

Smooth Endoplasmic Reticulum (SER)

—an irregular network of membrane-bounded channels, lacking ribosomes.

—usually appears in the form of branching anastomosing tubules and vesicles.

—serves different functions, depending on the cell type in which it is located; these include steroid hormone synthesis, drug detoxification, metabolism of lipid and cholesterol, and release and recapture of calcium ions during contraction and relaxation.

Mitochondria

—rod-shaped organelles just large enough to be seen in the light microscope (0.2 μm in smallest dimension).

—have a double-membrane structure.

—outer membrane surrounds the entire organelle; inner membrane infolds into the interior of the organelle to form cristae, which contain enzyme complexes of the electron-transport chain that function in oxidative phosphorylation.

—have a matrix (inner compartment) that contains matrix granules that bind divalent cations (Mg^{2+} and Ca^{2+}).

—have enzymes of the Krebs cycle and fatty acid oxidation located in their matrix.

—contain their own genetic apparatus composed of DNA (circular), mRNA, tRNA, and rRNA (with a limited coding capacity); most mitochondrial proteins are encoded for by nuclear DNA.

—produce adenosine triphosphate (ATP), the primary source of energy for the cell.

Golgi Apparatus (complex)

—consists of several disk-shaped saccules (cisternae) arranged in a stack.

—at one side of stack is an outer, convex (cis, forming) face.

—at other side of stack an inner, concave (trans, maturing) face.

—small vesicles (including transfer vesicles from the RER) are associated with the other (cis) face.

—condensing vacuoles (secretory materials becoming condensed into granules) are associated with the inner (trans) face.

—varies in size and development, depending on the type of cell in which it is located and the activity of the cell.

Functions

—include membrane recycling and redistribution; the synthesis of carbohydrates and lipoproteins; the modification of products through the addition of fatty acids, sulfation, and glycosylation, as well as the concentration and packaging of synthesized material into secretory granules.

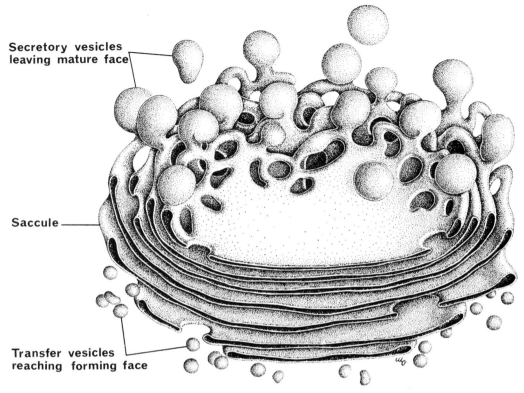

Secretory vesicles leaving mature face

Saccule

Transfer vesicles reaching forming face

Figure 1.2. Drawing of the Golgi apparatus. **Bottom,** the forming face with its transfer vesicles; **top,** the maturing face with its secretory vesicles. (From Ham AW, Cormack DH: *Histology*, ed 8. Philadelphia, JB Lippincott, 1979.)

Lysosomes
—membrane-bounded dense bodies approximately 0.2 to 0.5 μm in diameter.
—contain a number of hydrolytic enzymes that function in intracellular digestion.
—may be identified by their positive reaction to a cytochemical technique for acid phosphatase.

Primary Lysosomes
—newly released storage vesicles that have not yet engaged in digestive activity.

Secondary Lysosomes
—originate several ways, are sites of digestive activity, and include the following:

    —heterophagic vacuole: formed when material taken in from outside becomes sequestered in a phagocytic vacuole that fuses with a primary lysosome.

    —autophagic vacuole: originates when an organelle to be destroyed is enveloped by endoplasmic reticulum membranes that form a vacuole that fuses with a primary lysosome.

    —multivesicular body: forms when fluid taken into cell in tiny pinocytotic vesicles is enveloped by a membrane that forms a vacuole that fuses with a primary lysosome.

Residual Body

—a cytoplasmic inclusion (having great variation in appearance), which contains indigestible material.

GERL

—an acronym for Golgi-associated Endoplasmic Reticulum from which Lysosomes originate.
—located close to the maturing face of the Golgi apparatus and believed by some to constitute a distinct organelle involved in lysosome synthesis.
—components stain for acid phosphatase; thus hydrolases might move directly from their endoplasmic reticulum elements to primary lysosomes and bypass the Golgi apparatus.

Coated Vesicles

—involved in receptor-mediated uptake of specific molecules by the cell.
—form after specific macromolecules bind to plasma membrane receptors, which induces clustering of receptors and the formation of coated pits, which invaginate and detach, forming coated vesicles.
—also originate from the endoplasmic reticulum and Golgi apparatus.
—have a cytoplasmic surface coat that has the appearance of bristles (fuzz) due to the protein clathrin; clathrin forms a lattice-like basket structure that envelops the vesicle and is thought to prevent the fusion of coated vesicles with other membranous organelles.
—play a major role in recycling, as receptors and clathrin are returned to the plasma membrane.

Peroxisome (microbody)

—a membrane-bounded organelle that stains cytochemically for catalase, an enzyme that synthesizes and destroys hydrogen peroxide.
—also contains urate oxidase and D-amino acid oxidase.
—often bordered closely by a profile of smooth endoplasmic reticulum.
—may or may not contain a crystalline core or nucleoid; human peroxisomes do not contain a nucleoid.
—function includes the metabolism of hydrogen peroxide, cholesterol, and lipids and the breakdown of purines and pyrimidines.

Centrioles

—are involved in cell division.
—exist as a pair of short rods oriented at right angles to one another; the pair is called a diplosome.
—self-replicate prior to cell division, as each parent centriole forms a procentriole at right angles to itself.
—form the poles of the mitotic spindle where microtubules originate and/or converge.
—have a wall made up of nine tubular triplets (which resemble a pinwheel when the centriole is cross-sectioned; see Fig. 1.1).
—form basal bodies that give rise to cilia and flagella.

Cytoskeleton

—refers to the structural framework of the cell.
—components in the cytoplasm that maintain cell shape, stabilize cell attachments, underlie endocytosis and exocytosis, play a role in cell motility, etc.

—includes several filamentous structures: microtubules, microfilaments, intermediate filaments, and the microtrabecular lattice.

Microtubules
—straight structures, 25 nm in diameter and several micrometers in length.
—exist in two categories:

> —a labile population that exists free in the cytoplasm and polymerizes or depolymerizes, depending on temperature, pressure, drugs, etc.
> —a stable population that forms the walls of centrioles and the axonemes of cilia and flagella.

—have a wall 5 nm thick, which surrounds a lumen-like region, and is composed of 13 spirally arranged parallel protofilaments (linear polymers of α- and β-tubulin dimers).
—often terminate near centrioles in small dense bodies known as centriolar satellites.
—have proteins associated with their walls [microtubular-associated proteins (MAPS)] that function in polymerization and may also serve as stabilizing cross-links.
—during polymerization exhibit polarity, so that tubulin subunits are added at only one end (usually the end away from the initial site of nucleation).
—are associated with kinensin, a force-generating protein that may serve as a "motor" for organelle transport.
—function in maintaining cell shape, aid in the transport of macromolecules, and promote the movement of cilia, flagella, and chromosomes.

Actin Microfilaments (thin filaments)
—6-nm filaments (F-actin form) that comprise 10 to 15% of total cell protein; actin also exists in a globular form (G-actin).
—abundant in the periphery of the cell, where they form a dense meshwork beneath the plasma membrane.
—are involved in the sol-gel transformation of the cytoplasm, endocytosis, exocytosis, and the locomotion of nonmuscle cells.

Myosin Filaments (thick filaments)
—measure approximately 15 nm in diameter.
—are typically associated with actin in muscle cells.
—in striated muscle, are polymerized into clearly visible filaments.

Myosin
—also present in nonmuscle cells in low concentrations where its function is not well understood.
—exists in a variety of molecular sizes and configurations and can be induced to form bipolar filaments in vitro.

Intermediate Filaments
—a heterogeneous population measuring 8 to 11 nm in diameter.
—include keratin, vimentin, desmin, neurofilaments, and glial filaments.

Keratin Filaments (tonofilaments)
—characteristic of epithelial cells and are often associated with desmosomes.

Desmin Filaments

—in smooth, skeletal, and cardiac muscle form a framework that links myofibrils together.

Vimentin Filaments

—found in fibroblasts and other cells derived from mesenchyme.

—stabilize the nucleus and are closely associated with the nuclear envelope and nuclear pores.

Neurofilaments

—provide support for long processes of nerve cells and help to preserve the gel state of the cytoplasm.

Glial Filaments

—present in the nonneuronal cells of the central nervous system (astrocytes, oligodendrocytes, and microglia).

Microtrabecular Lattice

—a three-dimensional meshwork of slender strands existing in the ground substance of cells.

—has been identified in individual cells by use of the high-voltage electron microscope; its organization has been studied in only a few cells.

—demonstrates that the ground substance is not a homogeneous protein solution but a highly structured gel that links filamentous components and organelles into a single structural and functional unit (the cytoplast).

—thought to coordinate the metabolic activities of the cell by directing proteins to specific regions.

Inclusions

—lifeless accumulations of material within the cell.

—usually stored only temporarily.

—typically include glycogen, lipid droplets, and some secretion granules.

Glycogen

—a storage form of carbohydrate that varies in appearance at the ultrastructural level.

—may appear as electron-dense aggregates (known as the α-rosette arrangement) or as small clusters of β-particles.

—may also appear "unstained," if the method of tissue preparation has included en bloc treatment with uranyl acetate.

Lipid Droplets

—display different appearances depending on the fixation used (black with osmium; light gray with aldehydes).

—may or may not be limited by a membrane but typically have a homogeneous appearance.

Secretion Granules

—include mucous droplets, certain hormones, proteins, and pigment granules.

Cell Cycle

—cell may be described as having two major periods in its life cycle: interphase (the interval of nondivision) and mitosis (the interval of division).

—length of the cell cycle varies greatly in different types of cells, but with each cell generation the cycle is repeated.
—cells that no longer divide leave the cell cycle and are designated G_0 cells.

Interphase
—constitutes most of the cell cycle and is the major interval between successive mitoses.
—composed of three separate phases (G_1, S, G_2) where specific cellular functions take place.

G_1 Phase
—just after mitosis; a gap phase in which growth and protein synthesis occur.
—during this phase the daughter cell is restored to normal volume and size.

S Phase
—follows the G_1 phase and is the time when DNA and histone synthesis occur.
—centrioles are also self-duplicated in S phase.

G_2 Phase
—follows the S phase and extends up to mitosis.
—the cell is preparing to divide and centrioles (which have self-duplicated) are growing to maturity.
—energy production for the completion of mitosis is also taking place.

Mitosis
—is the time of cell division that follows the G_2 phase.
—completes the cell cycle.
—results in the production of two identical daughter cells.

Prophase
—begins when the chromosomes thicken and become rod-like.
—each chromosome can be seen to consist of two parallel chromatids attached to one another at a constricted region, the centromere.

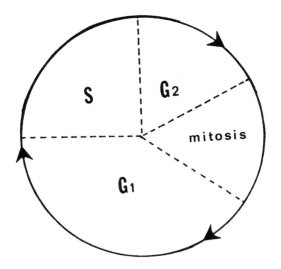

Figure 1.3. Diagram of the cell cycle, indicating gap 1 (G_1), synthesis (S), gap 2 (G_2), and mitosis.

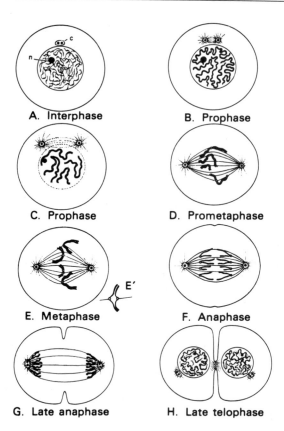

Figure 1.4. Diagram illustrating the phases of mitosis. **c**, Centrioles; **n**, nucleus; **E′**, enlargement of one of the metaphase chromosomes being pulled apart. (From Kelly DE, Wood RL, Enders AC: *Bailey's Textbook of Microscopic Anatomy*, ed 18. Baltimore, Williams & Wilkins, 1984.)

—associated with the disappearance of the nuclear envelope; by the end of prophase the nucleolus is no longer observed.

—centrioles (which have self-duplicated prior to prophase) migrate to opposite poles of the cell to form sites where the spindle fibers and the astral rays originate (both are composed of microtubules).

Metaphase

—occurs as the condensed chromosomes align themselves midway in the spindle at the equatorial plate.

—the kinetochore, which develops at the centromere region, is thought to play a role in this process, since it is an attachment site for the chromosomal microtubules of the spindle.

Anaphase

—begins as the chromatids separate at the centromere and daughter chromosomes move to opposite poles of the cell.

—associated with an elongation of the spindle.

—also characterized (in its later stages) by a furrow that begins to form around the cell to initiate cytoplasmic cleavage; this constriction furrow is the result of contraction by a band of actin filaments.

Telophase

—is characterized by a deepening of the cleavage furrow, which leaves an isthmus of material (the midbody) between the newly formed cells.

—associated with a depolymerization of microtubules in the midbody, which facilitates the completion of cytoplasmic cleavage and the formation of two identical daughter cells.

—includes reformation of the nuclear envelope around the condensed chromosomes in the daughter cells.

—associated with the reappearance of nucleoli, which form from specific nucleolar organizer regions on a few chromosomes, called secondary constriction sites.

—daughter nuclei gradually enlarge and the dense chromosomes disperse to form the typical interphase nucleus with heterochromatin and euchromatin.

REVIEW TESTS
THE CELL

DIRECTIONS: *One* or *more* of the given statements or completions is/are correct. Choose answer:

    A. if only **1**, **2**, and **3** are correct
    B. if only **1** and **3** are correct
    C. if only **2** and **4** are correct
    D. if only **4** is correct
    E. if **all** are correct

1.1. The plasma membrane
1. is associated with certain cytoskeletal components
2. consists of a lipid trilayer
3. contains a glycocalyx on its external surface
4. does not permit protein movement within the plane of the membrane

1.2. The nuclear pore
1. is hexagonal in shape
2. is bridged by a unit membrane
3. is a transient (rather than stable) structure
4. allows for communication betwen the nucleus and the cytoplasm

1.3. Ribosomes
1. are attached to the surface of the inner nuclear membrane
2. are organized into polysomes in cells synthesizing intracellular proteins
3. are always associated with a strand of mRNA
4. consist of a large and a small subunit

1.4. Smooth endoplasmic reticulum
1. often occurs in the form of branching, anastomosing tubules
2. sometimes has ribosomes attached to its membranes
3. is present in cells where drug detoxification is taking place
4. is rarely found in skeletal muscle cells

1.5. The Golgi apparatus
1. has condensing vacuoles associated with its outer (cis) face
2. has condensing vacuoles associated with its inner (trans) face
3. synthesizes multivesicular bodies
4. functions in the synthesis of certain lipoproteins

1.6. Intracellular digestion
1. is associated with lysosomes
2. includes the process of autophagy
3. is involved in the turnover of organelles
4. takes place within the Golgi apparatus

1.7. The cytoskeleton
1. includes microtubules
2. includes the microtrabecular lattice
3. includes intermediate filaments
4. includes actin filaments

1.8. Clathrin
1. forms part of the glycocalyx
2. plays a role in receptor-mediated uptake of specific molecules
3. is part of the cytoskeleton
4. makes up part of coated vesicles

DIRECTIONS: Select the *one* lettered structure on Figure 1.5 that best corresponds to the numbered word, phrase, or description listed below. Each letter may be used once, more than once, or not at all.

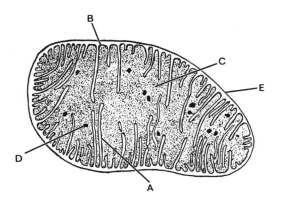

Figure 1.5. From Krause WJ, Cutts JH: *Concise Text of Histology*, ed 2. Baltimore, Williams & Wilkins, 1986.

1.9. contains enzymes of Krebs citric acid cycle

1.10. a crista

1.11. binds divalent cations

1.12. inner compartment

DIRECTIONS: Select the *one* lettered structure on Figure 1.6 that best corresponds to the numbered word, phrase, or description listed below. Each letter may be used once, more than once, or not at all.

1.13. inactive chromatin

1.14. location of fibrous (nuclear) lamina

1.15. site of rRNA synthesis

1.16. chromatin being transcribed

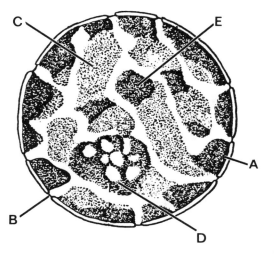

Figure 1.6. From Krause WJ, Cutts JH: *Concise Text of Histology*, ed 2. Baltimore, Williams & Wilkins, 1986.

DIRECTIONS: Each of the following statements contains five suggested completions. Choose the *one* that is *best* in each case.

1.17. The nuclear envelope

A. is not found in all epithelial cells
B. extends across nuclear pores
C. contains euchromatin
D. is formed by two nuclear membranes
E. is sometimes continuous with saccules of the Golgi apparatus

1.18. All of the following are inclusions (rather than organelles) *except*

A. a fat droplet
B. a lysosome
C. glycogen
D. a crystalloid
E. a mucous granule

1.19. The nucleolus is characterized by all of the following *except*

A. a fibrillar component representing early stages in the formation of ribosomal RNA (rRNA) precursors
B. nucleolar-associated chromatin
C. the nuclear lamina
D. a granular component representing late stages in the formation of rRNA precursors
E. the packaging of rRNA into precursors of ribosomes

1.20. All of the following are true of lysosomes *except*

A. they are associated with acid phosphatase activity
B. they function in intracellular digestion
C. they contain a number of hydrolytic enzymes
D. they can be identified by a cytochemical reaction for catalase
E. they often appear as membrane-bounded dense bodies

1.21. Mitosis in the cell cycle includes all of the following *except*

A. anaphase
B. prophase
C. metaphase
D. interphase
E. telophase

ANSWERS AND EXPLANATIONS

THE CELL

1.1. B (1 and 3)
Interactions between the plasma membrane and the cytoskeleton underlie many dynamic cell processes, such as endocytosis, maintenance of cell shape, and cell movement. The outer aspect of the lipid bilayer has a carbohydrate-rich glycocalyx, or cell coat. Certain plasma membrane proteins move within the plane of the membrane and thus change their location with time.

1.2. D (4)
Nuclear pores are complicated, octagonally shaped structures. They are bridged by eight radially arranged spokes and contain a dense central granule. The pores provide avenues of communication between the nucleus and cytoplasm, although the role played by the nuclear pore complex in allowing such passage of molecules in unknown.

1.3. C (2 and 4)
Cells synthesizing *secretory* proteins are characterized by an abundance of rough endoplasmic reticulum, since most of their ribosomes are attached to the endoplasmic reticulum (in the form of polyribosomes). Newly synthesized protein accumulates in the cisternae, then is packaged in the Golgi and is exported from the cell. In constrast, cells synthesizing protein for their *own use* have most of their ribosomes organized into polyribosomes that lie free in the cytoplasm. To synthesize protein, ribosomes need to associate with a molecule of mRNA; otherwise they are nonfunctional and lie free in the cytoplasm.

1.4. B (1 and 3)
Smooth endoplasmic reticulum may appear as vesicles, in addition to branching tubules. Since it does not have attached ribosomes it is "smooth." Cells involved in detoxification have large amounts of smooth endoplasmic reticulum and so does skeletal muscle (where it is specialized as the sarcoplasmic reticulum).

1.5. C (2 and 4)
The Golgi produces condensing vacuoles at its inner, trans face, and these are subsequently concentrated into secretory granules. The synthesis of carbohydrates and lipoproteins is among the functions of the Golgi apparatus.

1.6. A (1, 2, and 3)
The process of intracellular digestion involves the interaction of primary lysosomes with cytoplasmic vacuoles, into which the lysosomes release their hydrolytic enzymes. The intracellular degradation may involve organelles and parts of the cell (autophagy) or material taken from outside (heterophagy).

1.7. E (all are correct)
The structural framework of the cell, known as the cytoskeleton, is composed of several filamentous components: microtubules (25 nm), intermediate filaments (8 to 11 nm), microfilaments (6 nm), and a microtrabecular lattice.

1.8. C (2 and 4)
The selective (receptor-mediated) uptake of macromolecules by a cell occurs in coated pits that detach and form coated vesicles. The cytoplasmic coating of these structures consists of the protein clathrin, which forms a basket-like lattice encasement.

For questions **1.9** through **1.12**, refer to Figure 1.5.

1.9. C. Matrix.

1.10. A. Crista.

1.11. D. Matrix granule.

1.12. C. Inner compartment.

15

For questions **1.13** through **1.16**, refer to Figure 1.6.

1.13. **E.** Heterochromatin.

1.14. **A.** Fibrous nuclear lamina.

1.15. **D.** Nucleolus.

1.16. **C.** Euchromatin.

1.17. **D**

The nuclear envelope is formed by the inner and outer nuclear membranes and the narrow perinuclear space they envelop. It is present in all nucleated cells and is sometimes continuous with the endoplasmic reticulum.

1.18. **B**

A lysosome is considered to be an organelle, rather than an inclusion. It contains a number of hydrolytic enzymes and plays an active role in intracellular digestion. Inclusions are merely lifeless accumulations of material in the cytoplasm.

1.19. **C**

The nuclear lamina is a thin meshwork of filaments associated with the inner nuclear membrane. It serves as an anchoring site for interphase chromosomes.

1.20. **D**

The catalase cytochemical reaction identifies peroxisomes (microbodies), not lysosomes.

1.21. **D**

Mitosis does not include interphase, which is the interval between successive divisions.

2
Epithelium and Glands

Epithelium

—the tissue that lines the internal and covers the external surface of the body.
—specialized for different functions, such as absorption, secretion, transport, protection, etc.
—consists of one cell layer (simple epithlium) or more (stratified) arranged into sheets.
—has cells close to one another with little intercellular space.
—is avascular.
—composed of polarized epithelial cells, specialized to perform a variety of vectorial functions.
—separated from the underlying connective tissue by a filamentous layer, the basement membrane.

Glands

—have secretory portions composed of epithelial cells, which may secrete either into a duct (exocrine gland), into the bloodstream (endocrine gland), or into the extracellular space (paracrine gland).

Types of Epithelia
—classified into types by the number of cell layers and the shape of the superficial layer of cells.

Simple Squamous Epithelium
—consists of a single layer of flattened cells.
—lines blood vessels (as endothelium) and the pleural, peritoneal, and other serous cavities (as mesothelium).
—comprises the parietal layer of Bowman's capsule, the thin loop of Henle, etc.

Simple Cuboidal Epithelium
—consists of a single layer of polyhedral cells that appear cuboidal in histological sections.
—lines distal tubules in the kidney, follicles in the thyroid gland, the surface of the ovary, etc.

EPITHELIUM

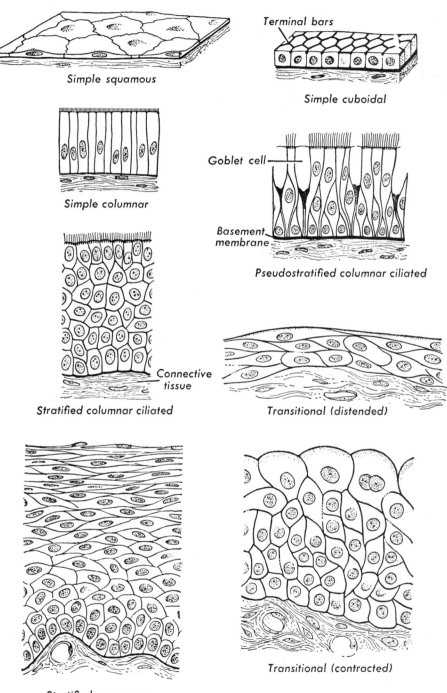

Figure 2.1. Diagram of the various types of epithelia with their basal laminae and underlying connective tissue. (From Kelly DE, Wood RL, Enders AC: *Bailey's Textbook of Microscopic Anatomy*, ed 18. Baltimore, Williams & Wilkins, 1984.)

Simple Columnar Epithelium
—consists of polyhedral cells, elongated in one plane, thus appear columnar in histological sections.
—cells are arranged in a single layer.
—lines the stomach, intestine, and the excretory ducts of many glands.

Stratified Squamous Nonkeratinized Epithelium
—composed of several layers of cells.
—the most superficial layer consists of flat nucleated cells.
—lines the moist body surfaces, such as the mouth, esophagus, vagina.

Stratified Squamous Keratinized Epithelium
—composed of several layers of cells.
—flattened superficial layers have lost their nuclei and become filled with keratin (become keratinized).
—constitutes the epidermis.

Stratified Cuboidal Epithelium
—composed of two or more layers of cells with the uppermost cells appearing cuboidal.
—lines the ducts of sweat glands but is otherwise uncommon.

Stratified Columnar Epithelium
—composed of two or more layers of cells, the most superficial being columnar in shape.
—relatively uncommon, but is occasionally found in the large excretory ducts of some glands and in the cavernous urethra.

Pseudostratified Epithelium
—falsely (pseudo)stratified, since every cell rests on the basal lamina but not all of them reach the lumen.
—lines the trachea, primary bronchi, excretory ducts in the parotid gland, etc.

Transitional Epithelium
—a stratified epithelium whose superficial cells (in the relaxed state) are dome-shaped and bulge into the lumen.
—when stretched, is reduced to only a few layers of flattened cells.
—undergoes marked changes in appearance, depending on the degree of stretch.
—lines excretory passages in the urinary system (from the renal calyces to the urethra).

Specializations of Epithelial Cell Surfaces

Lateral Surfaces

Junctional Complex
—a specialization found between epithelial cells that corresponds to the "terminal bar" observed in the light microscope.
—in electron micrographs can be seen to consist of three distinct components: the zonula occludens, zonula adherens, and macula adherens.

Zonula Occludens (tight junction)
—region where outer leaflets of adjacent plasma membranes fuse to form a zone around the entire apical perimeter of the cells.

—in freeze-fracture preparations, the en face view of this zone of fusion reveals a branching anastomosing network of intramembrane strands on the P face and grooves on the corresponding E face.

—complexity and number of strands (in apical to basal direction) determine the "leakiness" of the junction.

—prevents entrance, or exit, of substances into the intercellular space from the lumen.

Fasciae Occludentes

—analagous (ribbon-like) structures present in capillaries but do not extend around the entire cell.

Zonula Adherens (intermediate junction; belt desmosome)

—second component of the junctional complex.

—extends completely around the perimeter of the epithelial cells, just basal to the zonula occludens.

—plasma membranes in this zone are separated by 10 to 20 nm.

—opposing plasma membranes are reinforced on their cytoplasmic surfaces by a mat of actin filaments, which extend into the terminal web.

—intercellular space often contains an amorphous or filamentous material.

—an adhesive and structurally supportive junction.

Fasciae Adherentes

—analogous ribbon-like structures in the intercalated disks between cardiac muscle cells.

Macula Adherens (desmosome)

—third component of the junctional complex but also commonly found elsewhere attaching epithelial cells together.

—a focal, disk-shaped adhesive junction between adjacent epithelial cells.

—the adjacent cells are separated by a 15 to 30 nm space, and a dense plaque is present on the cytoplasmic surface of each of the opposing plasma membranes.

—intermediate (10-nm) keratin filaments (tonofilaments) from the cytoplasm loop into and out of the dense plaques.

—intercellular space between the two halves of the desmosome has dense material and delicate striations representing transmembrane linkers that are believed to assist in stabilizing this junction.

Gap Junction (nexus; communicating junction)

—a plaque-like specialization composed of an ordered array of subunits.

—not limited to epithelium but common between cells in the central nervous system, as well as between cardiac muscle and smooth muscle cells (where it was discovered and given the name "nexus").

—opposing plasma membranes remain separated by a 2 nm gap, which is bridged by connexons.

—each connexon consists of six cylindrical subunits (made up of the protein connexin) arranged radially around a central channel (1.5 nm diameter).

—connexons in the opposing plasma membranes extend into the intercellular "gap" and are aligned precisely so as to permit the passage of ions and small molecules (no greater than 1,200 MW) from cell to cell.

Lateral Interdigitations

—finger-like or irregular projections that interlock adjacent epithelial cells.

Basal Surface

Basal Lamina (basement lamina)

—an acellular supportive structure (20 to 100 nm thick) visible with the electron microscope and produced by the epithelium resting on it.

—composed mainly of Type IV collagen, laminin, and proteoglycans.

—consists of two zones: a low-density lamina rara (lamina lucida) lying next to the plasma membrane and a more dense meshwork of filaments (lamina densa) usually lying adjacent to the reticular lamina of the connective tissue.

—along with the reticular lamina comprises the "basement membrane" of light microscopy.

Hemidesmosome

—an attachment specialization that has the appearance of one-half of a desmosome.

—present along the basal surface of cells in certain epithelia, such as the basal cells in stratified squamous epithelia, myoepithelial cells in the mammary gland and salivary glands, and basal cells in the tracheal epithelium.

—attaches cells to the underlying basal lamina.

Basal Plasma Membrane Infoldings

—a common specialization in ion-transporting epithelia.

—form deep invaginations that compartmentalize mitochondria.

—ion pumps (Na^+-K^+-ATPase in the plasmalemma) are thus brought into close association with the energy supply (ATP from mitochondria).

Apical Surface

Microvilli

—finger-like projections of epithelium (approximately 1 μm in length) that extend into a lumen and increase the absorptive surface area.

—comprise the brush border of kidney proximal tubule cells and the striated border of intestinal absorptive cells.

—are characterized by a glycocalyx (sugar coat) on their exterior surface, which is formed primarily by the delicate branching terminal oligosaccharides of integral membrane proteins and phospholipids.

—contain a bundle of about 30 actin filaments (longitudinally arranged) that extend from the core of the microvillus into the terminal web of the apical cytoplasm.

Stereocilia

—are not cilia, but very long microvilli.

—present in the epididymis and vas deferens of the male reproductive tract.

Cilia

—actively motile specializations of certain epithelia (e.g., tracheobronchial epithelium, oviduct, etc.) that transport substances along their surfaces.

—measure 5 to 10 μm in length.

—are covered by a plasmalemma, and each cilium contains an axoneme, or core of longitudinal microtubules that has a constant number and precise arrangement; the axoneme consists of nine pairs of doublet tubules uniformly spaced around two single microtubules (9 + 2 pattern).

—from one of the doublet tubules two rows of arms project in a unidirectional fashion.

—the arms consist of dynein ATPase, which splits ATP to liberate energy necessary for the active movement of the cilium.

—at the base of each cilium is a cylindrical basal body, identical in structure to a centriole (having the 9 + 0 pattern of nine triplet microtubules radially arranged like a pinwheel).

Glandular Epithelium

Glands

—originate from lining epithelium that penetrates the connective tissue and forms secretory units.
—are of two major types: exocrine and endocrine.

Exocrine

—have ducts to convey material away from the secretory epithelium.

Endocrine

—lack ducts and release secretions into the bloodstream.
—secretory epithelial cells constitute the parenchyma of the gland, whereas connective tissue elements form its stroma.

Exocrine Gland

—classification is based on several parameters: the number of cells, the type of duct, the shape of the glandular unit, and the type and mode of secretion.

Unicellular

—a gland composed of a single cell (e.g., the goblet cell in tracheal epithelium).

Multicellular

—a gland composed of more than one cell.
—further classified into two subcategories, simple or compound, depending on whether or not the duct branches.

—simple gland: the duct does not branch.
—compound gland: the duct branches.

—shape of secretory unit defines whether the gland is classified as acinar or alveolar (sac- or flask-like) or tubular (either straight, coiled, or branched).

Architecture

—of a compound gland varies.
—some are surrounded by a connective tissue capsule; others have septa of connective tissue that divide the gland into lobes and smaller lobules.
—location of ducts in a gland may be interlobar (between lobes), or intralobar (within lobes), interlobular (between lobules), or intralobular (within lobules).

Type of Secretion

—may be classified as mucous, serous, or mixed:

—mucus is a viscous material produced by mucous glands that usually protects or lubricates.
—serous secretions (from serous glands) are watery and often rich in enzymes.

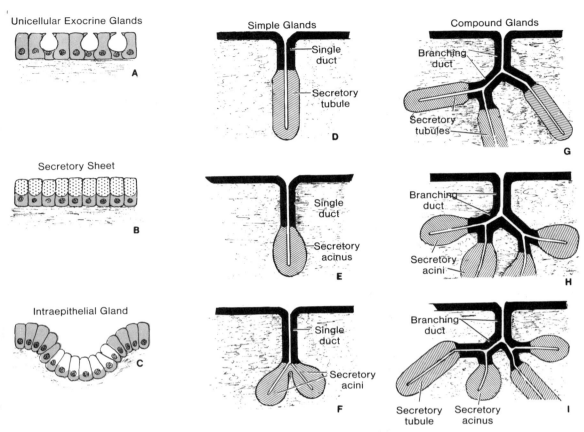

Figure 2.2. Diagram of various types of glands. **A**, unicellular glands; **B**, secretory sheet; **C**, intraepithelial gland; **D**, simple tubular gland; **E**, simple acinar gland; **F**, simple branched gland; **G**, compound tubular gland; **H**, compound acinar gland; **I**, compound tubuloacinar gland. (From Krause WJ, Cutts JH: *Concise Text of Histology*, ed 2. Baltimore, Williams & Wilkins, 1986.)

Method of Secretion

—may be merocrine, apocrine, or holocrine:

—merocrine mechanism is by exocytosis.
—apocrine is where part of the apical cytoplasm is released along with the secretory material.
—holocrine is where the entire cell and its contents are released.

Endocrine Gland

Classification

—may be unicellular, as the enteroendocrine cells in gastrointestinal and respiratory epithelia, or multicellular, when composed of more than one cell.

Characteristics

—include the lack of a duct system and release of hormone secretions into capillaries.
—a basal lamina separates the epithelium from the connective tissue compartment.
—blood vessels are abundant and may indent but do not penetrate the basal lamina.

REVIEW TESTS

EPITHELIUM AND GLANDS

DIRECTIONS: *One* or *more* of the given statements or completions is/are correct. Choose answer:

   A. if only **1**, **2**, and **3** are correct
   B. if only **1** and **3** are correct
   C. if only **2** and **4** are correct
   D. if only **4** is correct
   E. if **all** are correct

2.1. Which of the following characteristics are true of epithelia?
1. they line body surfaces
2. they are vascular
3. they are separated from underlying connective tissue by a basal lamina
4. they contain relatively large amounts of intercellular substance

2.2. The classical description of a junctional complex includes which of the following components?
1. the fascia occludens
2. the zonula adherens
3. the nexus
4. the zonula occludens

2.3. Microvilli
1. include stereocilia
2. form the brush border in proximal tubule cells of the kidney
3. facilitate absorption
4. contain an axoneme composed of 9 peripheral doublet microtubules and a central pair of microtubules

2.4. Centrioles
1. do not self-replicate
2. contain dynein arms that have ATPase activity
3. contain an inner core of actin filaments
4. contain a 9 + 0 configuration of microtubules

2.5. Gap junctions
1. permit the passage of large proteins from cell to cell
2. form part of the classical "junctional complex"
3. exist only between epithelial cells
4. exist as plaques made up of many connexons

2.6. The following statements are true regarding stratified squamous epithelium.
1. the surface layer of cells is always keratinized
2. it lines the esophagus
3. it lacks a basal lamina
4. its most superficial layer of cells is flattened

2.7. The desmosome
1. is a disk-like attachment between cells
2. is associated with keratin filaments
3. is specialized for adhesion
4. is located only between epithelial cells

24

DIRECTIONS: The following questions or statements refer to the electron micrograph (Fig. 2.3). Select the *one* lettered heading on the labeled electron micrograph that best corresponds to the numbered word, phrase, or description listed below. Each letter may be selected once, more than once, or not at all.

2.8. contains a core of actin filaments

2.9. keratin filaments (tonofilaments) converge upon it

2.10. the terminal web

2.11. the zonula occludens

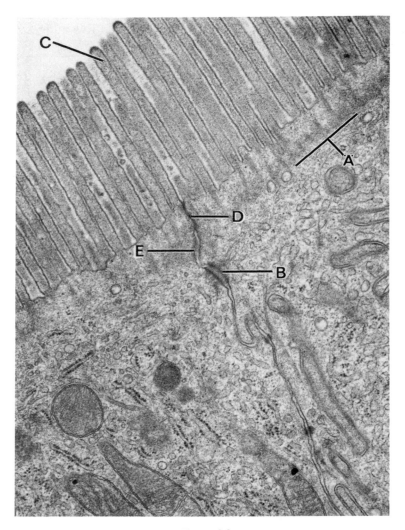

Figure 2.3.

DIRECTIONS: From the lettered headings below, select the *one* structure that is most closely associated with the numbered word:

A. axoneme
B. a core of actin filaments
C. 9 + 0 pattern of intermediate filaments
D. stereocilium
E. basal body

2.12. cilium

2.13. centriole

DIRECTIONS: Each of the following statements contains five suggested answers. Choose the *one* that is *best* in each case.

2.14. Simple squamous epithelium lines all of the following structures *except*

A. the alveoli of lungs
B. parietal layer of Bowman's capsule
C. lymphatic vessels
D. distal convoluted tubule
E. thin limb of Henle's loop

2.15. Centrioles are associated with each of the following *except*

A. ciliogenesis
B. nine triplet microtubules
C. dynein arms that possess ATPase activity
D. the ability to duplicate themselves
E. development of the mitotic spindle

2.16 In exocrine glands the intralobar ducts

A. are not present
B. lie within lobules
C. lie between lobules
D. lie within lobes
E. lie between lobes

ANSWERS AND EXPLANATIONS

EPITHELIUM AND GLANDS

2.1.   B (1 and 3)

Epithelia line the body cavities and surfaces. They are avascular tissues, since blood vessels do not penetrate the basal lamina but remain within the connective tissue compartment. Epithelial cells are joined tightly together via junctions and thus have little intercellular substance.

2.2.   C (2 and 4)

The junctional complex (as it was initially described in the intestinal epithelium) consists of the tight junction (zonula occludens), intermediate junction (zonula adherens), and desmosome (macula adherens). Although these three components are not always observed in all types of epithelia, the classical description of the junctional complex includes them.

2.3.   A (1, 2, and 3)

Microvilli form the brush border in proximal tubule cells and the striated border in intestinal epithelial cells where they provide an increased surface area for absorption. Stereocilia are very long microvilli. The core of each microvillus contains a number of actin filaments that extend into the terminal web region of the epithelial cell. The axoneme constitutes the core of a cilium.

2.4.   D (4)

Centrioles are identical in structure to basal bodies and give rise to cilia and flagella. Centrioles contain a complex internal arrangement of nine peripheral tubular triplets, a configuration known as the 9 + 0 pattern. A special feature of centrioles is that they are able to self-replicate.

2.5.   D (4)

Gap junctions permit the passage of ions and small molecules from cell to cell but exclude molecules greater than 1,200 MW. In addition to epithelial cells, these junctions exist between cardiac and smooth muscle cells and also between cells in the central nervous system. They are composed of a plaque made up of many connexons, each of which contains a central "channel" that regulates the passage of material from cytoplasm to cytoplasm.

2.6.   C (2 and 4)

Stratified squamous epithelium may be either keratinized or nonkeratinized (the latter lines the esophagus). It rests on a basal lamina, and its most superficial cells are flattened in shape.

2.7.   A (1, 2, and 3)

The desmosome is a disk-shaped junctional specialization found not only between epithelial cells but also between cardiac muscle cells. Its function is adhesion. Bundles of intermediate keratin filaments (tonofilaments) extend from the cytoplasm into and out of the cytoplasmic plaques that constitute part of the desmosome.

For questions **2.8** and **2.11**, refer to the electron micrograph, p. 25.

2.12.   A

The axoneme makes up most of the core of a cilium. It consists of microtubules arranged longitudinally into a precise (9 + 2) pattern that is a characteristic of cilia.

2.13.   E

A basal body appears identical to a centriole, but its precise function is to give rise to a cilium or a flagellum.

2.14.   D

The distal convoluted tubule is lined by a simple cuboidal epithelium, not a simple squamous epithelium.

2.15.   C

Centrioles do not possess dynein arms or ATPase activity. These are characteristics of cilia.

2.16.   D

The intralobar ducts lie *within* lobes of a gland [intra (within); inter (between)].

27

3

Connective Tissue

Connective Tissue

—consists of cells, fibers, and extracellular matrix material (ground substance).
—cell types are classified as "fixed" or "wandering."
—fibers may include collagen, reticular, or elastic fibers and are further classified according to size, morphology, and chemical composition.
—functions in support, as a medium for exchange between the blood and tissues, for storage, and for protection and repair.

Loose Connective Tissue

—possesses relatively fewer fibers but more cells and extracellular matrix than dense connective tissue.

Extracellular matrix

Composition

—includes glycosaminoglycans, proteoglycans, collagen, elastin, and the glycoproteins chondronectin, fibronectin, and laminin.
—matrix provides a medium for the transfer of nutrients and waste materials between connective tissue cells and the bloodstream.

Glycosaminoglycans (GAGS)

—linear polymers of disaccharides (one of which is always hexosamine). The major glycosominoglycans are hyaluronic acid, chondroitin sulfate, dermatan sulfate, keratan sulfate, and heparan sulfate.

Hyaluronic Acid

—is found in synovial fluid, vitreous humor, and most connective tissue proper.
—its huge domain permits it to act as a barrier to bacterial invasion.
—some pathogenic bateria may produce hyaluronidase, which liquifies hyaluronic acid and permits the spread of bacteria.

Chondroitin Sulfate

—is predominant in cartilage, bone, and the adventitia of large blood vessels. It is usually bound to a protein core.

Dermatan Sulfate

—is located mostly in skin, lung, and tendon.

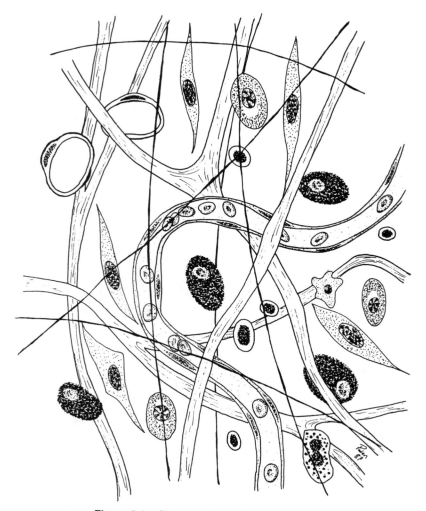

Figure 3.1. Diagram of loose (areolar) connective tissue.

Keratan Sulfate
—is found in the cornea, cartilage, and nucleus pulposus.

Heparan Sulfate
—is found in interalveolar septa in lung and in the connective tissue framework of the liver and aorta.

Proteoglycans
—consist of a core of fibrous protein to which glycosaminoglycans are covalently bound. Proteoglycans are attached to hyaluronic acid.

Glycoproteins
—include fibronectin, chondronectin, and laminin.
—possess a high proportion of protein and a variety of different polysaccharide side chains.

Fibronectin

—represents a group of closely related glycoproteins (MW = 440,000) found in connective tissue, basal laminae, and located on the surfaces of some cells.

—functions to bind cells to collagen and is involved in the aggregation of platelets and possibly in clot formation.

Plasma Fibronectin

—is located in the blood plasma, where it is thought to be synthesized by the endothelium.

—is synthesized also by several cell types, including fibroblasts, chondrocytes, myoblasts, Schwann cells, and a number of epithelia.

Laminin

—a large glycoprotein (MW = 440,000) found mostly in basal laminae, where it functions to attach epithelial cells to type IV collagen.

Fibers

Collagen

—the most abundant protein in the body, representing about 30% of the total body protein (dry weight).

—is a fibrous protein having great tensile strength that is composed of tropocollagen molecules.

—amino acids making up collagen are glycine (33.5%), proline (12%), and hydroxyproline (10%).

—fibroblasts manufacture and secrete procollagen (a precursor of tropocollagen) into the extracellular environment.

—procollagen has additional amino acids at the NH_2-terminal end of the molecule that are cleaved by the enzyme procollagen peptidase.

—tropocollagen molecules then self-assemble to form cross-striated fibrils of collagen (which must form covalent bonds to have tensile strength).

—electron micrographs reveal collagen fibrils to be 20 to 100 nm in diameter and display a cross-banding pattern. The major repeat period is every 64 to 67 nm, with sub-bandings in between.

Tropocollagen Molecules

—measure 280 nm in length and are composed of 3 polypeptide α-chains, each with MW = 100,000, entwined and cross-linked to form a rod-shaped molecule with a right-handed triple helix.

—self-assemble into parallel arrays overlapping each other by one-fourth of their length, leaving gaps between the NH_2-terminal end of one molecule and the COOH-terminal end of the next.

—heavy metals precipitate into these gaps and "stain" the molecule in this region; when viewed with the electron microscope, alternating light and dark bands (with a typical periodicity of 64 nm) are observed.

Types of Collagen

—Type I collagen is composed of two types of α-chains $[\alpha1(I)_2\alpha_2(I)]$ and is found in skin, bone, tendons and the cornea.

—Type II collagen is composed of three chains of of $[\alpha1(II)]_3$ and is found in cartilage.

—Type III collagen is composed of three identical $[\alpha1(III)]_3$ chains. This type constitutes reticular fibers and displays 64 nm banding.

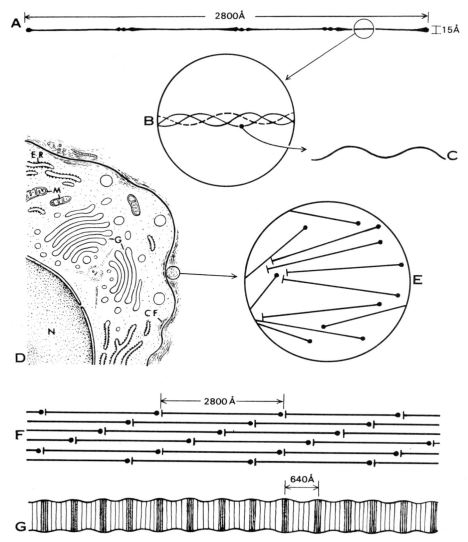

Figure 3.2. Diagram of collagen synthesis. **A**, tropocollagen molecule. **B**, the region within the circle (in **A**) is shown magnified, indicating that the three α-helices constitute the tropocollagen. **C**, enlargement of a section of the polypeptide chain, demonstrating its helical configuration. **D**, diagram of a region of a fibroblast with its organelles (**N**, nucleus; **M**, mitochondria; **G**, Golgi apparatus; **ER**, rough endoplasmic reticulum; **CF**, cytoplasmic filaments). **E**, enlargement of the unassembled tropocollagen molecules. **F**, schematic diagram of the proposed mode of assembly of the tropocollagen molecules to form collagen. **G**, diagram of the structure of collagen as seen in electron micrographs. (From Copenhaver WM, Kelly DE, Wood RL: *Bailey's Textbook of Histology*, ed 17. Baltimore, Williams & Wilkins, 1978.)

—Type IV collagen is composed of three identical $[\alpha 1(IV)]_3$ chains, is found in basal laminae, and does not display 64 nm banding.

—Type V collagen is composed of α-chains of undetermined composition and is found in basal laminae, fetal membranes, and blood vessels.

—Additional types of collagen are being identified but are outside of the purview of this book.

Recticular Fibers
—are thin fibers 0.5 to 2.0 μm in diameter; they consist mostly of Type III collagen and form networks of various organs and glands.
—stained by silver (they turn black) due to their high carbohydrate content.
—located in abundance in embryonic connective tissue and around fat and smooth muscle cells, as well as forming a fine supporting mesh in the liver, lymph nodes, and spleen.

Elastic Fibers
—are coiled, branching fibers 0.2 to 1.0 μm in diameter, which sometimes form loose networks.
—may be stretched up to 150% of their resting length.
—require special staining to be observed by light microscopy.
—electron micrographs display these fibers as microfibrils embedded in amorphous elastin.
—located in the dermis, lungs, elastic cartilage, ligamenta flava, and nuchae, as well as in large blood vessels, where they are arranged as cylindrical sheaths.

Cells

Fibroblasts
—the predominant cell of connective tissue that manufactures the precursors of the extracellular environment.
—fusiform, with long tapering ends when they are synthesizing; less-active fibroblasts may be flattened and possess several processes.
—nucleus is usually oval and often has two nucleoli.
—electron micrographs display more well-developed rough endoplasmic reticulum and Golgi in the active fibroblast than in the inactive cell.

Pericytes
—are smaller than fibroblasts but difficult to distinguish from them; this cell assumes the pluripotential role of the embryonic mesenchymal cell.
—are located mostly along capillaries.
—electron micrographs reveal coarse chromatin, few mitochondria, and very little rough endoplasmic reticulum.

Adipose Cells
—are responsible for the synthesis and storage of fat.
—types: unilocular and multilocular.

Unilocular Cells
—cytoplasm is squeezed to a thin rim around the periphery of the cell, with the flattened nucleus displaced to the rim to accommodate the fat droplet.
—form adipose tissue when present in large numbers.

Multilocular Cells
—contain many small fat droplets, and groups of these cells form brown fat.

Macrophages
—are the principal phagocytosing cells of the connective tissue responsible for removing particulate matter and assisting in the immune response.

—originate in the bone marrow, circulate in the bloodstream as monocytes, and migrate into the connective tissue, where they perform their major function.

—are spherical, 10 to 14 μm in diameter (when newly arrived), and possess a slightly basophilic cytoplasm.

—electron micrographs display a smooth cell contour with sparse endoplasmic reticulum and few inclusions.

—after activation the macrophages display filopodia, phagocytic vacuoles, secondary lysosomes, and residual bodies.

Foreign-Body Giant Cells

—are multinucleated masses of coalesced macrophages surrounding a foreign body.

Lymphocytes

—are cells that have migrated from the bloodstream into the connective tissue.

—types: T lymphocytes are responsible for initiating the cell-mediated immune response; B lymphocytes, when activated, differentiate to form plasma cells, which provide humoral immunity; and null cells, which have no surface determinants.

—located throughout the body in the subepithelial connective tissue. Accumulations of lymphocytes are found in the respiratory system, the gastrointestinal tract, and especially in areas of chronic inflammation. Their morphology is described in Chapter 5.

Plasma Cells

—are antibody-manufacturing cells that arise from activated B lymphocytes.

—are ovoid, contain an eccentrically placed nucleus, and possess clumps of heterochromatin that appear to be arranged in a spoke-wheel fashion.

—cytoplasm is deeply basophilic because of an abundance of rough endoplasmic reticulum. An area adjacent to the nucleus appears pale and contains the Golgi apparatus.

—electron micrographs display an extensive rough endoplasmic reticulum and a prominent Golgi apparatus reflecting the active protein synthesis occurring within their cells.

Eosinophils

—are white blood cells that have migrated from the blood into the connective tissue. They phagocytose Ab-Ag complexes and assist in destroying parasites. Their morphology is described in Chapter 5.

Mast Cells

—are found near small blood vessels. They possess a small, ovoid, pale-staining nucleus, and their cytoplasm is filled with coarse deeply stained metachromatic granules.

—electron micrographs reveal a surface possessing folds, a well-developed Golgi apparatus, little endoplasmic reticulum, and many dense lamellated granules.

—contain heparin, histamine, the slow-reacting substance of anaphylaxis, and eosinophil chemotactic factor.

—display IgE on their external plasma membrane and participate in anaphylactic reactions.

Dense Connective Tissue

—contains more fibers but less matrix and fewer cells when compared with loose connective tissue.

—fiber bundle arrangement determines whether classified as dense irregular or dense regular connective tissue.

Dense Irregular Connective Tissue

—comprises most dense connective tissue and is characteristic of the dermis and capsules of many organs.
—contains fibroblasts, mast cells, macrophages, and pericytes.

Dense Regular Connective Tissue

—includes only tendon and ligaments. The fibers are arranged in parallel bundles. The narrow spaces between groups of fibers are occupied by attenuated fibroblasts.

Special Connective Tissue

Mucous Connective Tissue

—a type of loose connective tissue found in the embryo (deep to the skin and in the umbilical cord).
—contains large stellate-shaped fibroblasts and a jelly-like matrix with some collagen fibers.

Embryonic Connective Tissue

—is composed of star-shaped, pale-staining mesenchymal cells embedded in a gel-like amorphous matrix containing only a few widely scattered fibers (mostly reticular).
—mitotic figures are frequently observed in these pluripotential mesenchymal cells.

Elastic Tissue

—coarse elastic fibers branching and rejoining with the spaces in between filled with a sparse network of collagen fibers and some fibroblasts.
—examples: ligamentum nuchae and the walls of the elastic vessels (where the elastic fibers form fenestrated sheets).

Reticular Connective Tissue

—bundles of thin, small collagenous fibers that blacken with silver.
—located around the liver sinusoids and forms the stroma of lymphatic organs. This tissue contains many free cells along with reticular cells.

Adipose Connective Tissue

—may be white (unilocular) or brown (multilocular)
—white adipose tissue: stores fat in large fat cells, is subdivided into lobes and lobules by thin sheaths of fibrous connective tissue, and has a rich neurovascular supply.
—capillary endothelium: possesses lipoprotein lipase, and enzyme that hydrolyses plasma lipoproteins and chylomicrons. The hydrolyzed fatty acids are released from the capillaries and enter the fat cells for storage and eventual release.
—brown adipose tissue: has a rich neurovascular supply. It is composed of multilocular adipose cells that contain numerous mitochondria, and is found mostly in infants as well as in animals that hibernate.
—produces heat by uncoupling oxidative phosphorylation.

REVIEW TESTS

CONNECTIVE TISSUE

DIRECTIONS: *One* or *more* of the given completions or answers is/are correct. Choose answer:

    A. if only **1, 2,** and **3** are correct
    B. if only **1** and **3** are correct
    C. if only **2** and **4** are correct
    D. if only **4** is correct
    E. if **all** are correct

3.1. Glycosaminoglycans
1. always contain hexosamine
2. include hyaluronic acid
3. are made up of disaccharides
4. are a primitive form of collagen

3.2. Which of the following statements regarding collagen is/are not true?
1. it is composed of tropocollagen
2. reticular fibers are composed of collagen
3. it possesses a 64- to 67-nm periodicity
4. elastic fibers are composed of collagen

3.3. Fibroblasts differentiate into
1. pericytes
2. macrophages
3. mast cells
4. none of the above

3.4. Glycoproteins found in the matrix include
1. laminin
2. chondronectin
3. fibronectin
4. dermatan sulfate

3.5. Mast cells possess or contain
1. heterochromatin arranged in a spoke-wheel pattern
2. deeply stained basophilic granules
3. well-developed endoplasmic reticulum
4. eosinophil chemotactic factor

DIRECTIONS: The following questions or statements refer to the photomicrograph (Fig. 3.3). The letters on the figure are answers to the numbered items appearing below the photomicrograph. For each numbered item select the *one* letter that *best* corresponds to that item. Each letter may be used once, more than once, or not at all.

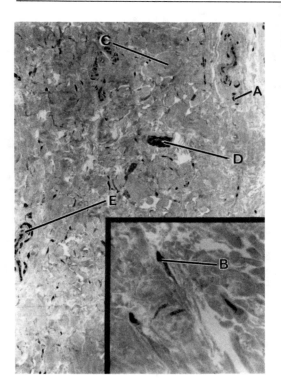

Figure 3.3. From Gartner LP, Hiatt JL: *Atlas of Histology*. Baltimore, Williams & Wilkins, 1987.

3.6. Identify the type of connective tissue.

3.7. Identify fibroblast.

3.8. Identify collagen bundle.

DIRECTIONS: Each of the following questions contains four suggested answers. Choose the *one best* response to each question.

3.9. Of the cell types found in connective tissue, which of the following is most often found along capillaries and resembles fibroblasts?

a. plasma cell
b. lymphocyte
c. macrophage
d. pericyte

3.10. Collagen precursors are secreted by

a. plasma cells
b. mast cells
c. fibroblasts
d. adipose cells

3.11. Dense regular connective tissue includes

a. organ capsules
b. basement mebranes
c. tendons
d. skin

3.12. Adipose cells

a. possess a flattened nucleus
b. possess a thin rim of cytoplasm
c. store fat
d. all of the above

3.13. Monocytes that circulate in the blood are the precursors of what cells in connective tissue?

a. plasma cells
b. fibroblasts
c. lymphocytes
d. macrophages

3.14. Foreign body giant cells are coalesced

a. macrophages
b. lymphocytes
c. fibroblasts
d. adipose cells

ANSWERS AND EXPLANATIONS

CONNECTIVE TISSUE

3.1. A (1, 2, and 3)
One of the characteristics of glycosamino-glycans is that one of its disaccharides is always hexosamine. Hyaluronic acid is also a glycosaminoglycan. Collagen is not made of glycosaminoglycans.

3.2. D (4)
Collagen is composed of tropocollagen molecules and possesses a periodicity of 64 to 67 nm. Reticular fibers are also composed of collagen, but elastic fibers are not. They are composed of elastin.

3.3. D (4)
Fibroblasts are completely differentiated cells and only revert to giving rise to other cells in pathological conditions.

3.4. A (1, 2, and 3)
Matrix glycoproteins include laminin, chondronectin, and fibronectin. Dermatan sulfate is a glycosaminoglycan.

3.5. C (2 and 4)
Mast cells possess a poorly developed endoplasmic reticulum, deeply stained basophilic granules, and in addition to heparin, histamine, and slow-reacting substance of anaphylaxis, they contain eosinophilic chemotactic factor. Plasma cells possess heterochromatin arranged in a spoked-wheel fashion.

3.6. Dense irregular collagenous connective tissue

3.7. Fibroblast **(B)**

3.8. Collagen bundle **(C)**

3.9. d
Pericytes are pluripotential cells that resemble fibroblasts, though they are smaller and located adjacent to capillaries. Plasma cells, macrophages, and lymphocytes are morphologically distinct from fibroblasts.

3.10. c
Collagen precursors are secreted by fibroblasts, which are responsible also for secreting the connective tissue matrix.

3.11. c
The tendon possesses an array of collagen fibers arranged in a regular ordered fashion.

3.12. d
Adipose cells, because of storing fat, have their cytoplasm and nucleus squeezed to a thin rim at the periphery of the cell.

3.13. d
Bloodborne monocytes leave the bloodstream and migrate into the connective tissue to become macrophages.

3.14. a
Foreign-body giant cells result when macrophages coalesce. Lymphocytes, fibroblasts, and adipose cells do not coalesce or form foreign-body giant cells.

4

Cartilage and Bone

Cartilage and Bone

—are specialized types of connective tissues, each of which has a unique matrix, fiber population, and characteristic cells.
—matrix of cartilage is firm but pliable.
—matrix of bone is calcified and forms the skeleton in higher vertebrates.
—both bone and cartilage function in support, but bone also serves as a reservoir for calcium and phosphate, protects vital organs, and contains bone marrow, which functions in hemopoiesis.

Cartilage

Hyaline Cartilage

Matrix

—is composed of amorphous ground substance and Type II collagen fibrils.
—collagen constitutes about 40% of the total matrix; is not discernible in histologic sections because the fibrils are very fine and have the same refractive index as the matrix.
—capsular matrix (matrix adjacent to the chondrocyte) is poor in collagen but rich in glycosaminoglycans.
—stains deeply basophilic. It is also metachromatic and stains more intensely with periodic acid–Schiff reaction (PAS) than other areas of the matrix.

Perichondrium

—is a connective tissue region surrounding cartilage, except at articular surfaces.
—composed of an outer fibrous layer containing Type I collagen, fibroblasts, and blood vessels and an inner cellular (chondrogenic) layer composed of chondrogenic cells.

Chondrogenic Cells

—in the inner layer of the perichondrium differentiate into chondroblasts, the cells that produce cartilage.

Chondrocytes

—are matured chondroblasts located in the lacunae of cartilage and are surrounded by matrix.
—located superficially, chondrocytes are ovoid and positioned so that their longitudinal axes lie parallel to the cartilage surface.
—located deeper, they are more spherical.

—isogenous groups (groups of four to eight cells) found in young cartilage are suggestive of interstitial growth.

—electron micrographs display irregular chondrocyte surfaces with some small processes. They also display an extensive Golgi apparatus, have an abundant rough endoplasmic reticulum, and contain lipid droplets and glycogen deposits.

Histophysiology

—Chondrocytes manufacture the matrix through which nutrients and waste materials pass to and from the cells via diffusion.

—hormones influence the growth of cartilage: thyroxine, testosterone, and growth hormone increase the growth rate; cortisone, hydrocortisone, and estradiol decrease it.

Histogenesis

—in the embryo, mesenchymal cells differentiate into chondroblasts. These basophilic cells secrete matrix and become incarcerated by it, thus becoming chondrocytes.

—interstitial growth (growth from within) occurs only in young cartilage from cell divisions within the cartilage.

—appositional growth occurs from chondrogenic cells in the perichondrium differentiating into chondroblasts, forming a new layer of cartilage around the periphery of the existing cartilage.

Regressive Change

—hyaline cartilage undergoes regressive changes. The cells hypertrophy and die and the matrix becomes calcified.

—some of these changes also occur in the process by which cartilage participates in endochondral bone formation.

Regeneration

—hyaline cartilage regenerates very poorly and often the perichondrium forms scar tissue.

Location

—hyaline cartilage is the most common cartilage in the body. It is found at the articular ends of long bones; in the nose, larynx, trachea, and the bronchi; and it serves as the skeleton of the fetus.

Elastic Cartilage

—is often found with hyaline cartilage. It possesses a perichondrium, grows by apposition, and does not degenerate as readily as hyaline cartilage.

—located where support with flexibility is required, as in the ear, auditory tube, and epiglottis.

—matrix is identical to that of hyaline cartilage, except it also contains a network of elastic fibers that impart to it a yellowish color.

Fibrocartilage

—is associated with the capsules and ligaments of joints.

—serves as a transition between connective tissue and cartilage, as in the annulus fibrosus of the intervertebral disks.

—does not occur alone, but is found in conjunction with hyaline cartilage and other fibrous tissues.

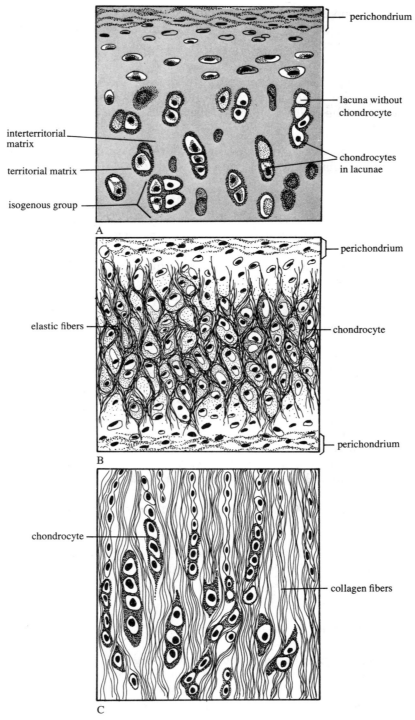

Figure 4.1. Diagram of the three types of cartilages. **A**, hyaline cartilage. **B**, elastic cartilage. **C**, fibrocartilage. (From Borysenko M, Berringer T: *Functional Histology*, ed 2. Boston: Little and Brown, 1984.)

—located where support and tensile strength is of utmost importance, such as in the intervertebral disks, articular disks, pubic symphysis, and at the insertions of some tendons and ligaments.

Matrix
—is composed of Type I collagen, chondroitin sulfate, and dermatan sulfate.
—collagen fiber bundles are arranged parallel to the stress placed on the cartilage, and chondrocytes lie in longitudinally disposed columns between them.

Fibroblasts
—of the dense collagenous connective tissue differentiate into chondrocytes in regions of stress and transform the tissue into fibrocartilage.

Bone

—is composed of a calcified matrix and contains osteogenic cells, osteoblasts, osteocytes, and osteoclasts.
—osteogenic cells differentiate into osteoblasts, which secrete the organic matrix that entraps these cells.
—osteocytes (are entrapped) lie in cavities called lacunae.
—osteoclasts are multinucleated giant cells derived from monocytes responsible for resorbing and remodeling bone.

Matrix
—organic portion is composed of about 95% Type I collagen and amorphous ground substance.
—contains chondroitin 4-sulfate, chondroitin 6-sulfate, and keratan sulfate in addition to osteomucoid (a protein differing from collagen in that it does not contain hydroxyproline, has only a small amount of proline and glycine, but an abundance of tyrosine and leucine).
—inorganic portion represents about 50% of the dry weight of the matrix and is composed of calcium, phosphorus, bicarbonate, citrate, magnesium, potassium, and sodium.
—hydroxyapatite crystals $Ca_{10}(PO_4)_6(OH)_2$ are formed of calcium and phosphorus.

Vascular Supply
—blood vessels entering the periosteum and endosteum penetrate the bone matrix via Volkmann's canals, which run perpendicularly to the haversian canals that they interconnect.

Periosteum
—is a noncalcified connective tissue layer covering bone on its external surfaces, except at articular regions.
—is composed of an outer, fibrous and an inner, cellular layer: outer layer consists mostly of a dense collagenous connective tissue containing blood vessels; inner layer is more cellular and contains osteogenic cells and osteoblasts.
—Sharpey's fibers (collagen fibers of the periosteum that penetrate the bone matrix) function in attaching the periosteum to bone.
—functions to provide a blood supply to bone and is a source of osteogenic cells.

Endosteum
—is a specialized connective tissue lining the marrow cavities of bone.
—contains the same elements as the periosteum but is thinner and composed of osteogenic cells and osteoblasts.
—supplies osteogenic cells and osteoblasts for growth and repair.

Bone Cells

Osteogenic Cells
—are spindle-shaped connective tissue cells (derived from embryonic mesenchyme) in the periosteum and endosteum that are capable of differentiating into osteoblasts.
—low O_2 tension may cause these cells to change into chondrogenic cells.

Osteoblasts
—are derived from osteogenic cells; are basophilic.
—on bone surface may resemble a cuboidal layer as they commence secreting organic matrix. Later as matrix synthesis declines they assume a flattened morphology.
—contain cytoplasmic processes that bring them into close contact with other osteoblasts and osteocytes.
—electron micrographs reveal that during synthesis the osteoblast has a well-developed rough endoplasmic reticulum and Golgi apparatus.
—PAS-positive granules in the cytoplasm are most likely the precursors of glycosaminoglycans (of the osteoid matrix).
—matrix secretion entraps the osteoblast in a lacuna with its cytoplasmic processes extending into canaliculi to maintain contact with other cells. Ceasing its secretory function, it changes its morphology and becomes an osteocyte.

Osteocytes
—are derived from osteoblasts. These mature bone cells, housed in their own lacunae, maintain communication with each other via gap junctions between their narrow cytoplasmic processes extending through the canaliculi.
—nutrients and metabolites within canaliculi nourish and maintain these cells.
—electron micrographs display increased amounts of condensed nuclear chromatin, reduced amounts of rough endoplasmic reticulum, and a small Golgi apparatus.

Osteoclasts
—are multinucleated giant cells (possessing as many as 50 nuclei) that are thought to result from the fusion of blood-derived monocytes.
—Howship's lacunae are depressions located on the bone surface that house osteoclasts. These lacunae result from the osteolytic activities of osteoclasts.
—electron micrographs display four regions: ruffled border, clear zone, vesicular region, and basal region.

Ruffled Border
—is composed of finger-like evaginations along Howship's lacunae. Active bone resorption occurs here.

Clear Zone
—is the region of cytoplasm that surrounds the ruffled border.
—contains microfilaments, which are believed to assist the osteoclast in maintaining contact with the bony surface and isolating the region of osteoclastic activity.

Vesicular Region

—is composed of polymorphous vesicle-like structures that presumably depict the extracellular spaces between the finger-like evaginations of the ruffled border.

Basal Region

—houses the organelles and the numerous nuclei of the osteoclast.

Function

—osteolysis, by creating an acidic environment that decalcifies the surface bone layer; then acid hydrolases, collagenases, and proteolytic enzymes degrade decalcified material and the cell resorbs the organic and inorganic residues of the bone matrix.

Types and Classification

Compact Bone

—is very dense and mature.

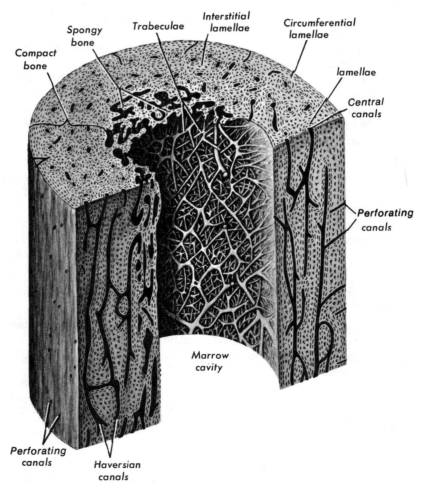

Figure 4.2. Diagram of the diaphysis of a long bone. (From Kelly DE, Wood RL, Enders AC: *Bailey's Textbook of Microscopic Anatomy*, ed 18. Baltimore, Williams & Wilkins, 1984.)

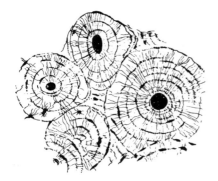

Figure 4.3. Diagram of an osteon and interstitial lamellae. (From *Stedman's Medical Dictionary*, ed 24. Baltimore, Williams & Wilkins, 1984.)

Spongy Bone
—is filled with spaces that are interconnected. These spaces in long bones often contain bone marrow, which may be either red (containing hemopoietic cells) or yellow (containing primarily fat).

Primary Bone
—immature or woven bone; the first compact bone elaborated; contains large populations of osteocytes and irregularly arranged collagen and possesses a low-mineral content.
—is remodeled and replaced by secondary bone, except in certain places such as in tooth sockets, near suture lines in the bones of the skull, and at insertion sites of tendons.

Secondary Bone
—(mature or lamellar bone) has haversian systems, or osteons. This bone replaces primary bone and is the compact bone of adults.
—calcified matrix is arranged in regular concentric layers, or lamellae, (3 to 7 μm thick) surrounding a haversian canal that transmits blood vessels, nerves, and some loose connective tissue.
—osteocytes in lacunae are located between the lamellae and occasionally within them.
—cementing substance composed of an amorphous material is often observed between adjacent haversian systems.

Haversian System or Osteon
—is cylindrical and composed of 4 to 20 concentric lamellae. Because bone is constantly being remodeled, the haversian systems are not all in parallel array.
—lamellae exhibit a special arrangement in the diaphysis: there are outer circumferential lamellae and inner circumferential lamellae, as well as typical haversian systems, and interstitial (intermediate) systems.
—Volkmann's canals are the communication channels between haversian systems, between haversian canals and the periosteum, and between haversian canals and the marrow cavity.

Histogenesis
—bone develops in one of two ways: intramembranous bone formation involves development within a layer of condensed mesenchyme; endochondral bone formation occurs via a cartilage model that is replaced by bone.
—primary bone forms first and is later replaced by secondary bone.

—remodeling continues throughout life, although it is slower in secondary than in primary bone.

Intramembranous Bone Formation

—begins when mesenchymal cells condense to form a primary ossification center, from which osteoblasts differentiate and begin secreting osteoid.

—osteoblasts become trapped in their own matrix and become osteocytes.

—bony trabeculae (fused spicules) is the name given to the bone developing at these sites.

—spongy bone develops as bony trabeculae join together. Blood vessels invade the area at the same time that undifferentiated mesenchymal cells give rise to bone marrow cells.

—ossification centers fuse together, forming bone.

—examples of bone formed in this fashion include most of the flat bones of the skull.

Endochondral Bone Formation

—begins in a hyaline cartilage model.

Primary Center of Ossification

—occurs at the midriff of the diaphysis of the cartilage model.

—vascularization of the perichondrium at the midriff of the cartilage model causes the transformation of chondrogenic cells to osteogenic cells, which in turn differentiate into osteoblasts.

—osteoblasts elaborate bone matrix on the cartilage core beneath the perichondrium (now known as the periosteum). The new bone is the subperiosteal bone collar and is formed by intramembranous bone formation.

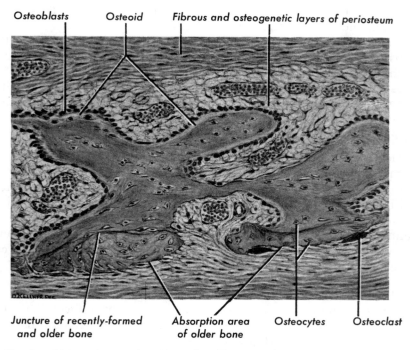

Figure 4.4. Drawing of intramebranous bone formation. (From Kelly DE, Wood RL, Enders AC: *Bailey's Textbook of Microscopic Anatomy*, ed 18. Baltimore, Williams & Wilkins, 1984.

—chondrocytes within the cartilage model hypertrophy and begin to degenerate; the lacunae become confluent and form spaces within the core of the cartilage model.
—osteoclasts etch holes in the bone collar, permitting the periosteal bud (osteogenic cells and blood vessels) to penetrate the cartilage model.
—calcification of the walls of the empty lacunae is followed by elaboration and calcification of bone matrix on the surface of calcified cartilage, forming a calcified cartilage–calcified bone complex.
—in histologic sections the calcified cartilage stains basophilic, while the calcified bone stains acidophilic.
—subperiosteal bone collar becomes thicker and elongates toward the epiphyses.
—osteoclasts begin to resorb the calcified cartilage–calcified bone complex, thus establishing the primitive marrow cavity.
—sequence of events recurs and spreads toward the epiphyses.

Secondary Center of Ossification
—occurs at the epiphyses. The sequence of events is similar to but not identical with the processes ocurring at the primary center.
—ossification beings as osteogenic cells from the blood and adjacent periosteum invade the epiphyses and differentiate into osteoblasts that elaborate bone matrix to replace the disintegrating cartilage.
—remaining cartilage now possesses two areas: an articular surface (that will remain through life) and the epiphyseal plate (that will be replaced by bone when growth ceases).
—epiphyseal plate continues to grow by adding new cartilage at the epiphyseal end while it is being replaced by bone at the diaphyseal end.
—diaphyseal bone becomes continuous with epiphyseal bone (connecting the two marrow cavities) at about 20 years of age, as the epiphyseal plate ceases to grow and is replaced.

Epiphyseal Plate
—contains five histologically distinctive zones. Beginning with the epiphyseal side of the plate they are as follows:

  —zone of reserve cartilage: cartilage with small, randomly arranged inactive chondrocytes.
  —zone of cell proliferation: rapid mitotic divisions give rise to rows of isogenous cell groups.
  —zone of cell maturation and hypertrophy: the chondrocytes are greatly enlarged and contain glycogen, and the cartilage matrix between neighboring cells becomes thin.
  —zone of calcifying cartilage: lacunae become confluent and the remnants of interlacunar matrices become calcified, causing chondrocytic death.
  —zone of provisional ossification: bone is beginning to be elaborated upon the calcified cartilage, and osteolytic activity begins to resorb the calcified bone–calcified cartilage complex.

Bone Repair
—fractured bone demonstrates damage to the bone matrix and bone cells in the region, as well as to the blood vessels supplying the area.
—hemorrhaging is followed by blood clotting, and macrophages remove much of the debris via phagocytosis.

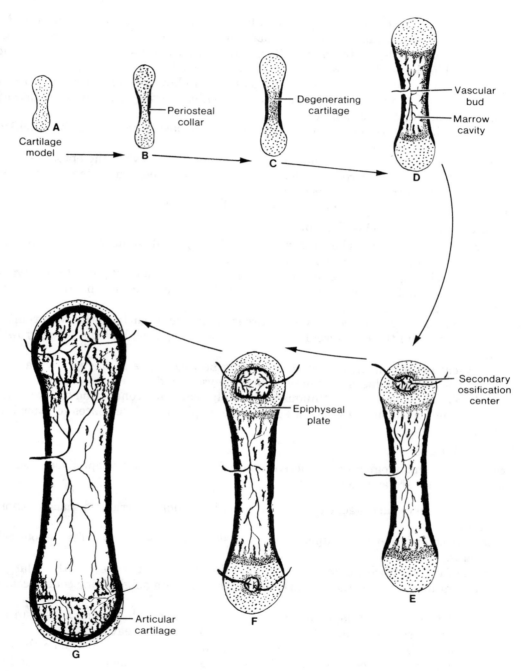

Figure 4.5. Diagram of endochondral bone formation. **A–G**, successive stages of this process. (From Krause WJ, Cutts JH: *Concise Text of Histology*, ed 2. Baltimore, Williams & Wilkins, 1986.

—fibroblasts proliferate in the periosteum and endosteum and surround the area internally and externally to isolate that area.

Callus
—is formed both internally and externally. Initially it is composed of bone and cartilage.
—bone is elaborated in the fracture zone via intramembranous bone formation by osteoblasts derived from osteogenic layer of the periosteum and endosteum in the vicinity of the fracture.
—chondrocytes also differentiate from this connective tissue and elaborate cartilage, which will be replaced by bone via endochondral bone formation, thus forming a bony callus composed of primary bone.
—bony callus is eventually resorbed and replaced with secondary bone as the repair process continues.

Histophysiology

Bone
—serves as a support for the body and provides for attachment of muscles. It also protects the central nervous system and vital organs.
—is dynamic tissue that constantly undergoes changes in shape and form because of the stresses placed upon it.
—growth is directed toward the applied stresses, while resorption takes place where pressures are applied.

Calcium Reserve
—bone is an important calcium reserve, containing about 99% of the body's calcium, an element essential for muscle contraction, enzymatic activities, transmission of nerve impulses, cell adhesion, and blood coagulation.
—decalcification of bone results from diet inadequate in calcium.
—during the remodeling of spongy bone, calcium is transferred from the bone into the bloodstream.

Nutrition
—greatly affects bone development. Diets low in protein result in a deficiency of amino acids essential for collagen synthesis by osteoblasts.
—lack of calcium, either from a low intake or inadequate absorption by the small intestine (due to a lack of vitamin D), results in poorly calcified bone, which leads to rickets in children and osteomalacia in adults.
—vitamin D is also necessary for ossification, and hypervitaminosis D causes bone resorption.
—vitamin A deficiency inhibits proper bone formation and growth, while excessive amounts of vitamin A accelerate the ossification of the epiphyseal plates. In either case, smaller stature results.
—vitamin C is necessary for collagen formation; its deficiency results in scurvy, characterized by poor bone growth and inadequate repair after fractures.

Hormones
—exert an influence on bone.

Parathyroid Hormone
—activates osteoclasts that resorb and release calcium, thus elevating blood calcium levels.

—may activate osteocytes to initiate osteolytic osteolysis, whereby they liberate calcium from the walls of their lacunae, thus elevating blood calcium levels.

—in excess renders bone more susceptible to fracture and subsequent deposition of calcium in arterial walls and certain organs such as the kidney.

Calcitonin

—inhibits matrix resorption and thus prevents the release of calcium.

Pituitary Growth Hormone

—stimulates epiphyseal cartilage growth, so that an excess produces a giant, while a lack produces a dwarf.

—acromegaly, a disease characterized by very thick long bones in adults as a result of an excess of growth hormone.

Sex Hormones

—affect bone growth by influencing epiphyseal ossification. In excess, a small stature develops; in deficiencies, a tall stature results.

Joints

Synarthroses

—are joints that are immovable. They may be composed of connective tissue, cartilage, or bone.

Diarthrosis

—are joints that permit maximum freedom of movement. They are synovial joints that are surrounded by a capsule.

—capsule (two layered) encloses and seals the synovial cavity about the joint: fibrous layer of capsule is the tough outer layer; synovial membrane is the inner more cellular layer composed of a layer of squamous-to-cuboidal cells that secrete the synovial fluid, a colorless viscous fluid, rich in hyaluronic acid and proteins.

—electron micrographs of the synovial membrane reveal two cell types that may be different physiological expressions of the same cell type; both may be phagocytic.

—type A cells are intensely phagocytic and display a well-developed Golgi apparatus, many lysosomes, and sparse rough endoplasmic reticulum.

—type B cells are very electron dense and exhibit a well-developed rough endoplasmic reticulum.

REVIEW TESTS

CARTILAGE AND BONE

DIRECTIONS: *One* or *more* of the given completions or answers is/are correct. Choose answer:

    A. if only **1, 2,** and **3** are correct
    B. if only **1** and **3** are correct
    C. if only **2** and **4** are correct
    D. if only **4** is correct
    E. if **all** are correct

4.1. Osteoclasts
1. are multinucleated cells
2. produce proteolytic enzymes
3. are found occupying Howship's lacunae
4. are derived from fibroblasts

4.2. Periosteum functions in
1. facilitating the nutrition of new bone
2. the production of osteoblasts
3. appositional bone growth
4. initiating bone repair

4.3. Osteocytes
1. communicate with each other via canaliculi
2. live only for a short time
3. possess long narrow cytoplasmic processes
4. give rise to osteoclasts

4.4. Hyaline cartilage
1. is a vascular structure
2. contains Type II collagen
3. grows by interstitial growth only
4. plays a role in endochondral bone formation

4.5. Bone grows
1. not at all
2. only interstitially
3. by two methods
4. only appositionally

4.6. Periosteal buds
1. invade the cartilage model in endochondral bone formation
2. carry blood vessels and osteogenic cells
3. are involved in laying down primary bone
4. develop into periosteum

4.7. Volkmann's canals
1. contain no blood vessels
2. are arranged perpendicularly to the bone surface
3. are at the center of the osteon
4. communicate with haversian canals

4.8. Bone
1. is a storehouse for calcium
2. is depleted of collagen during calcification
3. is vascular
4. is not influenced by sex hormones

4.9. The following are true as regards bone and nutrition:
1. vitamin C is essential for collagen synthesis
2. osteomalacia is related to a lack of vitamin A
3. lack of vitamin D causes poor calcification
4. hypervitaminosis A produces bone resorption

4.10. Synovial membranes
1. are lined with squamous-to-cuboidal cells that secrete synovial fluid
2. produce hyaluronic acid
3. contain A and B cells
4. are found in diarthrosis joints

DIRECTIONS: The following questions or statements refer to the photomicrograph (Fig. 4.6). The letters on the figure are answers to the numbered items appearing below the photomicrograph. For each numbered item, select the *one* letter that *best* corresponds to that item. Each letter may be used once, more than once, or not at all.

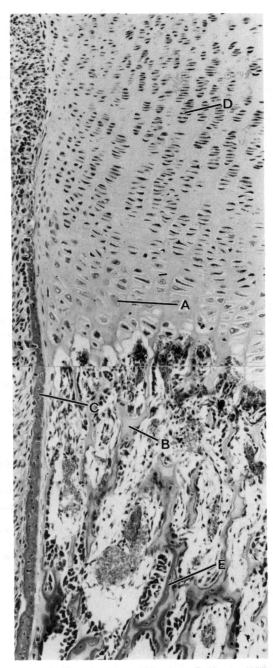

Figure 4.6. From Gartner LP, Hiatt JL: *Atlas of Histology*. Baltimore, Williams & Wilkins, 1987.

4.11. subperiosteal bone collar

4.12. zone of proliferation

4.13. calcified cartilage–calcified bone complex

4.14. zone of calcifying cartilage

4.15. zone of maturation and hypertrophy

ANSWERS AND EXPLANATIONS

CARTILAGE AND BONE

4.1. A (1, 2, and 3)
Osteoclasts are multinucleated cells that produce proteolytic enzymes and occupy Howship's lacunae. They are derived from monocytes, not fibroblasts.

4.2. E (all answers)
The periosteum functions to provide nutrition to the new bone via its vascularity. It also produces osteoblasts, which produce new bone by appositional growth. Repairing bone is also a function of this important structure.

4.3. B (1 and 3)
Osteocytes communicate with each other via narrow cytoplasmic processes that extend through canaliculi. They do not, however, give rise to osteoclasts, and they usually live for a long time as they maintain the structure of bone.

4.4. C (2 and 4)
Hyaline cartilage contains Type II collagen and plays a role in endochondral bone formation. It grows interstitially and appositionally and is avascular.

4.5. D (4 only)
Bone grows continually and by apposition only, unlike cartilage, which grows by two methods.

4.6. A (1, 2, and 3)
Periosteal buds carry blood vessels and osteogenic cells into the cartilage model in endochondral bone formation. These buds are then responsible for giving rise to cells that produce primary bone.

4.7. C (2 and 4)
Volkmann's canals are arranged at an angle perpendicular to the bone surface. They contain blood vessels and communicate with vessels in the haversian canal. The haversian blood vessels are located in the center of osteons.

4.8. B (1 and 3)
Bone is a highly vascular tissue that serves as a depository for calcium. Sex hormones influence ossification in the epiphyseal plate. Since collagen forms the organic portion of bone, it is not depleted during ossification.

4.9. A (1, 2, and 3)
Vitamin C is essential for collagen formation, and vitamin D is required for proper calcification. A deficiency of vitamin A causes osteomalacia, while an excess of this vitamin accelerates ossification of the epiphyseal plates, resulting in a small stature.

4.10. E (all answers)
Synovial membranes are lined with squamous-to-cuboidal cells that are derived from mesenchyme. They contain both A and B cells, which secrete synovial fluid that is rich in hyaluronic acid.

4.11. Subperiosteal bone collar (**C**)

4.12. Zone of proliferation (**D**)

4.13. Calcified cartilage–calcified bone complex (**E**)

4.14. Zone of calcifying cartilage (**B**)

4.15. Zone of maturation and hypertrophy (**A**)

5
Blood and Hemopoiesis

Blood

—a specialized type of connective tissue, is composed of formed elements (cells and platelets), suspended in a fluid intercellular material, known as plasma.
—volume in an average adult person is approximately 5 liters.
—circulates throughout the body in a closed system of vessels, transporting various nutrients, waste products, hormones, proteins (such as γ-globulins), electrolytes, etc.
—also regulates body temperature and assists in the regulation of osmotic and acid-base balance.
—circulating blood cells have a relatively short life span; they must be replaced continuously. Hemopoiesis is the process of new blood cell formation from stem cells.

Plasma

Composition
—90% water, 9% organic compounds (proteins, amino acids, hormones, etc.), and 1% inorganic salts.

Plasma Proteins
—are fibrinogen, albumin, and globulins.

Fibrinogen
—is converted into fibrin during the process of clotting by the action of various blood-borne enzymes and cofactors.

Albumin
—a small protein (60,000 MW), functions in preserving the osmotic pressure within the vascular system and in transporting certain metabolites.

Globulins
—are of three types, α, β, and γ.
—γ-globulins are antibodies utilized in immunological defense.
—α- and β-globulins transport metal ions (such as iron and copper) and lipids (in the form of lipoproteins).

Serum

—is the yellowish fluid remaining after blood has clotted. It is similar in composition to plasma but lacks fibrinogen and other clotting factors.

Formed Elements

Erythrocytes

Morphology

—round, biconcave disks, 7 to 8 μm in diameter, which stain light salmon pink with Wright's or Giemsa's modifications of the Romanovsky type stains. Mature red blood cells (RBC) lack nuclei.

Number

—$5 \times 10^6/mm^3$ in males; $4.5 \times 10^6/mm^3$ in females.

Life Span

—approximately 120 days in the circulation.

Blood Groups

—the determinants for the A, B, and O blood groups reside on the external surface of the erythrocyte plasma membrane.

Peripheral Proteins

—are associated with the internal aspect of the cell membrane. Those of major significance are protein 4.1, ankyrin, spectrin, and actin.

—spectrin and actin help maintain the shape of the RBC, while protein 4.1 and ankyrin bind actin and spectrin to the integral proteins on the cytoplasmic surface of the plasma membrane.

Ultrastructure

—neither organelles nor nuclei are present in the mature erythrocyte.

Hemoglobin

—is composed of four polypeptide chains, each covalently linked to a heme group (modified porphyrin ring).

—types of normal hemoglobin in the human adult depend on the amino acid sequences of the polypeptide chains and are known as Hb A_1, Hb A_2, and Hb F (fetal hemoglobin).

—predominant group is Hb A_1. Additionally, abnormal hemoglobin, such as Hb S, may also be present in the population.

—Hb S is the result of a point mutation (glutamate for valine) that causes sickling of the red blood cells (sickle cell anemia).

Energy Production

—since erythrocytes do not possess mitochondria, their energy requirements are met by the presence of soluble enzymes responsible for glycolysis and the hexose monophosphate shunt.

Function

—in the transport of oxygen and carbon dioxide to and from tissues of the body.

—in regions of high partial pressure of oxygen, hemoglobin preferentially picks up oxygen to form oxyhemoglobin.

—in regions of high partial pressure of carbon dioxide, oxyhemoglobin releases its oxygen, exchanging it for carbon dioxide, to form carboxyhemoglobin.

Carbon Monoxide
—also binds to the hemoglobin molecule, but its bond is much more tenacious than that of oxygen.

Leukocytes

—leukocytes (white blood cells; WBC) are subdivided into two groups, granulocytes and agranulocytes, depending on the presence or absence of specific granules in their cytoplasm.
—number in peripheral blood varies from 6500 to 9000/mm^3.
—granulocytes are neutrophils, eosinophils, and basophils.
—agranulocytes are lymphocytes and monocytes.

Neutrophils

Morphology
—round cells, 9 to 12 μm in diameter, whose dark blue nucleus presents a lobulated appearance (usually 3 to 4 lobes connected to each other by thin threads of chromatin).

Barr Body (sex chromosome)
—a drumstick-like evagination protruding from the nucleus that is seen in females. It is one of the two X chromosomes in an inactive state.

Cytoplasm
—of neutrophils stains light pink and displays occasional azurophilic and many fine specific granules.

Number
—3500 to 7000/mm^3 (60 to 70% of all leukocytes).

Life Span
—less than 1 week.

Ultrastructure
—reveals a small, centrally located Golgi apparatus, sparse rough endoplasmic reticulum, few mitochondria, and occasional free ribosomes.
—primary lysosomes (referred to as azurophilic granules) are well represented and glycogen is plentiful.

Specific Granules
—do not stain well. They are small (0.1 μm diameter), mostly spherical, and in electron micrographs they appear to be bounded by a membrane.
—contents of these granules are lysozyme, phagocytin, collagenase, and alkaline phosphatase.

Azurophilic Granules
—are primarily lysosomes that are fewer in number but are considerably larger than specific granules (approximately 0.5 μm diameter).
—contain various hydrolytic enzymes that function in phagocytosis. Fusion between

Table 5.1.
Formed Elements of Blood[a]

	Erythrocyte	Lymphocyte	Monocyte	Neutrophil	Eosinophil	Basophil	Platelets
Diameter							
Smear	7–8 μm	8–10 μm	12–15 μm	9–12 μm	10–14 μm	8–10 μm	2–4 μm
Section	6–7 μm	7–8 μm	10–12 μm	8–9 μm	9–11 μm	7–8 μm	1–3 μm
No./mm³	5×10^6 males 4.5×10^6 females	1,500–2,500	200–800	3,500–7,000	150–400	50–100	250,000–400,000
% of leukocytes		20–25	3–8	60–70	2–4	0.5–1	
Granules	None	Azurophilic only	Azurophilic only	Azurophilic and small specific (neutrophilic)	Azurophilic and large specific (eosinophilic)	Azurophilic and large specific (basophilic) granules (heparin and histamine)	Granulomere
Function	Transport of O_2 and CO_2	Immunologic response	Phagocytosis	Phagocytosis	Phagocytosis of antigen-antibody complexes and control of parasitic diseases	Perhaps phagocytosis	Agglutination and clotting
Nucleus	None	Large, round, acentric	Large, kidney-shaped	Polymorphous	Bilobed (sausage-shaped)	Large S-shaped	None

[a]From Gartner LP, Hiatt JL: *Atlas of Histology*. Baltimore, Williams & Wilkins, 1987.

azurophilic granules and phagosomes occurs subsequent to fusion of specific granules with phagosomes.

Function of Neutrophils

—avidly phagocytic. These cells migrate from the bloodstream between endothelial cells (diapedesis) to enter the connective tissue spaces, to form the first line of defense during acute inflammation.

—recognize and phagocytose bacteria.

—specific granules then fuse with the phagosome, whose pH is now decreased.

Azurophilic Granules

—fuse with the vacuole, releasing their hydrolytic enzymes into it, digesting the microorganism and ultimately killing the neutrophil.

Pus

—is the accumulation of dead neutrophils, macrophages, microorganisms, and tissue fluid.

Eosinophils

Morphology

—round cells, 10 to 14 μm in diameter.

Nucleus

—is brownish black and bilobed, resembling a pair of linked sausages.

Cytoplasm

—is obscured because of the many specific granules that stain reddish orange. Azurophilic granules are also present.

Number

—150 to 400/mm^3 (2 to 4% of all leukocytes).

Life Span

—less than 2 weeks in connective tissue.

Ultrastructure

—relatively few organelles, although mitochondria, a Golgi apparatus, and rough endoplasmic reticulum are present.

—glycogen deposits are plentiful, and a few azurophilic granules are also observed.

Specific Granules

—large, ellipsoidal, membrane-bounded, refractile granules (0.5 to 1.5 μm long; 0.3 to 1 μm wide).

—electron micrographs depict an elongated crystalline core surrounded by a flocculent to homogeneous material.

—contents: lysosomal enzymes, a peroxidase, and major basic protein (an arginine-rich component of the crystalline core that inactivates histamine).

Azurophilic Granules

—0.5 μm in diameter, are present in small numbers. They contain acid phosphatase, arylsulfatase, and other hydrolytic enzymes.

Function

—is not known conclusively, although eosinophils are believed to phagocytose antibody-antigen complexes, and they are also implicated in inactivating and killing parasitic agents.

—eosinophils respond to eosinophilic chemotactic factor and inactivate histamine and the slow-reacting substance of anaphylaxis (SRS-A), all of which are released by mast cells and basophils.

Allergic Reactions

—cause an increase in the eosinophil population, whereas hydrocortisone decreases the number of bloodborne eosinophils.

Basophils

Morphology

—are round cells, 8 to 10 μm in diameter, whose light blue S-shaped nucleus is frequently masked by the numerous dark, large specific granules. Azurophilic granules are also present.

Number

—the least numerous of all blood cells, 50 to 100/mm³ (0.5 to 1% of all leukocytes).

Life Span

—probably very long; in mice it is 1 to 1.5 years.

Ultrastructure

—a relatively sparse number of organelles, although mitochondria, a Golgi apparatus, and rough endoplasmic reticulum are all represented.

—contents: specific granules, a moderate amount of glycogen, and a few azurophilic granules.

Specific Granules

—are large (0.5 to 1.3 μm diameter) membrane-bounded, spherical structures containing granular particles in a homogeneous to flocculent matrix.

—contents: heparin, histamine, a peroxidase, and perhaps SRS-A.

Azurophilic Granules

—are lysosomes. They are few in number and contain hydrolytic enzymes.

Function

—similar to mast cells, in that basophils release histamine, heparin, SRS-A, and eosinophil chemotactic factor. They are mildly phagocytic.

Plasmalemma

—external aspect contains IgE receptors. When these receptors bind specific antigens, the basophils degranulate to produce cell-mediated immunity and, in extremely severe cases, anaphylactic shock.

Monocytes

Morphology

—the largest of all circulating cells, 12 to 15 μm in diameter.

Nucleus

—is acentric, kidney-shaped (usually lobated), displaying a coarse heterochromatin network intermingled with clear spaces representing heterochromatin. Usually two nucleoli are present.

Cytoplasm

—is grayish blue, containing numerous azurophilic granules. Since this is an agranulocyte, specific granules are not present.

Number

—200 to 800/mm^3 (3 to 8% of all leukocytes).

Life Span

—probably less than 3 days in the bloodstream.

Ultrastructure

—a prominent Golgi apparatus but relatively sparse rough endoplasmic reticulum, few mitochondria, and some ribosomes. Azurophilic granules and glycogen are evident, as are microfilaments and microtubules. Filopodia, pinocytotic vesicles, and phagosomes are also apparent.

Azurophilic Granules

—are quite numerous. They are primary lysosomes (0.5 μm diameter), containing peroxidase, acid phosphatase, and arylsulfatase, among other enzymes.

Function

—monocytes migrate into connective tissue, where they differentiate into macrophages and phagocytose particulate matter. They also process antigens in some unknown manner so as to facilitate antibody production by immunocompetent cells.

Lymphocytes

Morphology

—spherical, small cells, 8 to 10 μm in diameter, whose deeply staining, acentric nucleus occupies most of the cell, leaving a narrow rim of light blue cytoplasm at the periphery.

Medium and Large Lymphocytes

—(up to 18 μm diameter) are present in lymphatic organs and are believed to be T or B lymphocytes that are in the process of responding to an antigenic challenge by differentiating into lymphoblasts.

Azurophilic Granules

—are also present in the lymphocyte cytoplasm.

Number

—next to largest population of white blood cells, 1500 to 2500/mm^3 (20 to 25% of all leukocytes).

Life Span

—T lymphocytes may live for several years, whereas B lymphocytes die within a few months.

Ultrastructure

—small lymphocytes possess a few mitochondria, a poorly developed Golgi apparatus, hardly any rough endoplasmic reticulum, but an abundant supply of free ribosomes. A few lysosomes (azurophilic granules, 0.5 μm diameter) are also present.

Categories of Small Lymphocytes

—there are two types of lymphocytes: T lymphocytes and B lymphocytes.

—classification is according to their specific surface determinants and their site of differentiation.

—null cells, a third group, possessing no surface determinants, may also be demonstrated.

Function

—T lymphocytes are primarily responsible for cell-mediated immunity, whereas B lymphocytes provide humoral immunity.

Subgroups

—of T and B lymphocytes have different functions (these are discussed in Chapter 9, Lymphatic Tissue).

—null cells have at least two categories: undifferentiated totipotential hemopoietic stem cells that are responsible for hemopoiesis, and natural killer (NK) and killer (K) cells, which are cytotoxic cells that do not require potentiation by the thymus.

Platelets

Morphology

—round-to-oval cell fragments derived from megakaryocytes in the bone marrow. Platelets measure 2 to 4 μm in diameter, display a peripheral clear region (the hyalomere), and a more dense, granular center (the granulomere).

Number

—250,000 to 400,000/mm^3.

Life Span

—less than 2 weeks.

Ultrastructure

—a small bundle of microtubules lies just deep to the plasmalemma and encircles the periphery of the platelet, maintaining its oval morphology.

Hyalomere

—contains actin filaments, a surface-opening (connecting) tubular system, and a dense tubular system (which probably functions in sequestering calcium ions).

Granulomere

—is composed of α-granules (300 to 500 nm diameter), dense bodies (250 to 300 nm diameter), occasional mitochondria, a few lysosomes, and clusters of glycogen particles.

Glycocalyx

—composed of glycosaminoglycans and glycoproteins, coats the plasmalemma. In the presence of calcium ions and ADP it facilitates stickiness of the platelets so that, if needed, they may adhere to each other and to the vessel wall.

α-Granules

—contain fibrinogen, platelet thromboplastin, and growth factor.

Dense Bodies

—contain pyrophosphate, ADP, ATP, serotonin, and calcium.

Function

—coagulation of blood by their aggregation and involvement in clot formation.

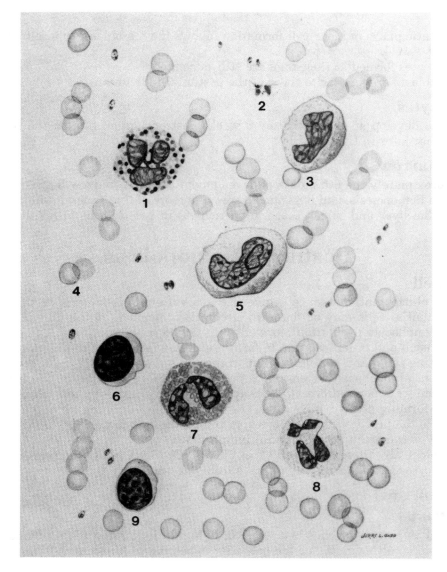

Figure 5.1. Diagram of circulating blood. **1**, basophil; **2**, platelets; **3**, monocyte; **4**, erythrocyte; **5**, monocyte; **6**, lymphocyte; **7**, eosinophil; **8**, neutrophil; **9**, lymphocyte. (From Gartner LP, Hiatt JL: *Atlas of Histology*. Baltimore, Williams & Wilkins, 1987.)

Prenatal Hemopoiesis

Yolk Sac

—hemopoiesis begins at 2 weeks postconception via the formation of blood islands in the yolk sac mesoderm (mesoblastic phase).

—mesoderm cells develop into large primitive erythroblasts that give rise to nucleated erythrocytes; however, at this stage no leukocytes are formed.

Liver
—the hepatic phase of blood cell formation follows the mesoblastic phase by approximately 4 weeks.
—erythrocytes formed at this stage are still nucleated.
—erythroblasts are similar to those of the postnatal individual.

Leukocytes
—begin to develop at approximately 8 weeks postconception, first in the liver and somewhat later in the spleen.

Bone Marrow
—in approximately the 6th month of development the bone marrow begins to participate in hemopoiesis, and it assumes more and more of that function shortly thereafter. The liver and spleen cease to participate in hemopoiesis about the time of birth.

Postnatal Hemopoiesis

Stem Cells
—toti- or pluripotential stem cells give rise to a variety of cells found in the blood.
—pluripotential cells may be found in circulation (members of the null cells of the small lymphocyte population), as well as in the bone marrow.
—cell division and differentiation to form precursors for each of the various types of circulating cells (and platelets) occur in the bone marrow.
—totipotential hemopoietic stem cell population (THSC) gives rise to two pluripotential stem cell populations, CFU-S (colony-forming unit—spleen) and CFU-Ly (colony-forming unit—lymphocyte).
—CFU-S is the precursor of monocytes, granulocytes, and platelets.
—CFU-Ly is the precursor of T and B lymphocytes.
—morphologically these three cell types (THSC, CFU-S, CFU-Ly) appear similar to lymphocytes and are indistinguishable from one another.

Bone Marrow

Yellow Marrow
—is found in the long bones of adults. It is highly infiltrated with fat and is not hemopoietic (although it has the potential to become so if necessary).

Red Marrow
—is found in the epiphyses of long bones, as well as in flat, irregular, and short bones.
—composed of a highly vascular tissue, housing large venous sinusoids, stromal cells, and many islands of hemopoietic cells.
—sinusoids are large (45 to 80 μm diameter) vascular channels with a highly attenuated endothelial lining.
—extravascular surfaces of sinusoids are associated with reticular fibers and the adventitial reticular cells that manufacture them.

Adventitial Reticular Cells
—are believed by some to subdivide the bone marrow cavity into smaller compartments, which are occupied by islands of hemopoietic cells.
—possibly adventitial reticular cells, rather than adipose cells, accumulate fat and transform red marrow into yellow marrow.

Macrophages

—are located in the extravascular areas near the sinusoids and extend their processes between the endothelial cells into the sinusoidal lumina.

Stem Cells

THSC

—a totipotential stem cell that gives rise to two groups of pluripotential stem cells: CFU-Ly and CFU-S.

CFU-Ly

—a pluripotential (immunoincompetent) stem cell that is responsible for the formation of B and T lymphocytes, as well as the NK and K cells of the null cell population.

CFU-S

—a pluripotential stem cell (colony-forming unit—spleen) that resembles a small lymphocyte (null cell) that possesses no surface determinants.

—cytoplasm contains only a few mitochondria and free ribosomes.

—nucleus presents an undifferentiated appearance in that it has little heterochromatin.

—descendants of this cell are presented in Table 5.2. CFUs derived from this cell (with the exception of more CFU-S) are either unipotential or possess the ability to give rise to two cell lines.

Erythrocyte Formation

BFU-E

—(burst-forming unit—erythropoietic) are committed cells, derived from CFU-S, that have tremendous rates of mitotic activity and give rise to a large number of CFU-E.

—respond to high concentrations of erythropoietin (a hormone produced by the kidneys that stimulates erythropoiesis).

CFU-E

—committed cells, arising from BFU-E, that respond to low concentrations of erythropoietin. They are the immediate precursors of the first histologically recognizable erythrocyte precursor, the proerythroblast.

Proerythroblast

—the largest of the erythrocytic series (14 to 19 μm diameter).

—nucleus is large, round, centrally placed, burgundy red, and displays a fine chromatin network. Three to five pale gray nucleoli are usually apparent.

—cytoplasm is a pale gray blue that exhibits deep blue clumps of material.

—electron micrographs demonstrate the presence of ferritin in the cytoplasm. Proerythroblasts divide to produce the next cell in the erythrocytic series.

Basophilic Erythroblast

—is smaller (12 to 17 μm diameter), and its nucleus resembles that of the proerythroblast, except that the chromatin network is coarser and nucleoli may not be present.

—cytoplasm also appears similar, with markedly basophilic clumps in a slightly grayish pink background.

—electron micrographs reveal abundant free ribosomes, some mitochondria, a few

**Table 5.2.
Hemopoiesis**

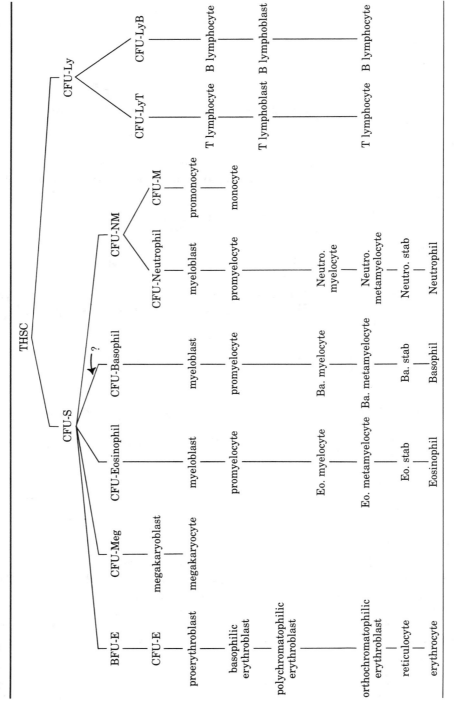

profiles of rough endoplasmic reticulum, and a Golgi apparatus. The cytoplasm also contains some hemoglobin, recognizable as homogeneous, electron-dense deposits.

Polychromatophilic Erythroblast

—arises from division of the basophilic erythroblasts. It is 12 to 15 μm in diameter and has a round, densely staining nucleus that demonstrates a coarse chromatin network.

—cytoplasm presents a yellowish pink hue (indicative of a large amount of hemoglobin being synthesized) interspersed in a blue background. Organelles are decreased in number, and this is the last stage where cell division occurs.

Orthochromatophilic Erythroblast (normoblast)

—a small cell (8 to 12 μm diameter) with a dark, condensed, pyknotic nucleus that may be in the process of being extruded from the cell or may be located eccentrically.

—extruded nucleus, surrounded by a thin rim of cytoplasm, is usually phagocytosed by resident macrophages.

—cytoplasm is pink with a trace of blue, and in electron micrographs displays a few mitochondria and ribosomes, with large quantities of electron-dense hemoglobin.

Reticulocyte

—lacks a nucleus and may be slightly larger than erythrocytes but cannot be differentiated from them unless stained with supravital dyes, such as cresyl violet or methylene blue, to display a reticulum.

—reticulum is dark blue, composed of rough endoplasmic reticulum and polysomes.

—pseudopodial migration is the process whereby the reticulocyte leaves the bone marrow through the endothelial lining of the sinusoids.

—ubiquitin is the enzyme that destroys the remaining organelles within 3 days of arriving in the bloodstream, afterwhich the cell becomes a mature erythrocyte.

Number

—of erythrocytes produced daily by a normal adult is estimated to be over 1 trillion.

Granulocytic Series

Granulocytes

—are of three types, each of which is derived from its own (uni- or bipotential) stem cell population, a descendant of the CFU-S: CFU-Eo (Eo, eosinophils), CFU-NM [which gives rise to neutrophils and monocytes (NM)], and possibly CFU-B (the precursor of basophils).

—produce the histologically recognizable myeloblast, which is the progenitor of granulocytes.

Neutrophil Formation

Myeloblast

—12 to 14 μm in diameter; a large round reddish blue nucleus exhibits a fine chromatin network. Two or three pale gray nucleoli are evident.

—cytoplasm displays blue clumps in a pale blue background and has no granules. The periphery of the cell is frequently marked by the presence of filopodia-like cytoplasmic blebs.

—electron micrographs demonstrate the presence of rough endoplasmic reticulum, a small Golgi apparatus, numerous mitochondria, and many free ribosomes.

Promyelocyte

—is larger than the myeloblast (16 to 24 μm diameter). The nucleus of the promyelocyte displays a coarse chromatin network and possesses one or two nucleoli.

—cytoplasm reveals a bluish hue and contains numerous azurophilic granules. The periphery of the cell no longer displays filopodia-like cytoplasmic blebs.

—electron micrographs demonstrate the presence of a well-developed Golgi apparatus, rough endoplasmic reticulum, and numerous mitochondria.

—azurophilic granules, approximately 0.5 μm in diameter, form from the maturing face of the Golgi apparatus. They are lysosomes that contain hydrolytic enzymes and peroxidase.

Neutrophilic Myelocyte

—10 to 12 μm in diameter; a somewhat flattened acentric nucleus displays a coarse chromatin network. A nucleolus may or may not be observed.

Specific Granules

—(0.1 μm diameter; contain lysozyme, alkaline phosphatase, collagenase, and phagocytin) are clearly evident, as are the azurophilic granules noted in the previous stage.

Golgi Apparatus

—displayed as a clear area, is also conspicuous in the pale blue cytoplasm.

—electron micrographs demonstrate the presence of a well-developed Golgi apparatus.

—specific neutrophilic granules are derived from the forming face of the Golgi apparatus. The significance, if any, of this derivation is not known.

—cell division still occurs, and it is the only stage where specific neutrophilic granules are formed.

Neutrophilic Metamyelocyte

—is similar to the neutrophilic myelocyte, except that its nucleus is kidney shaped and displays a coarse chromatin network that lacks nucleoli.

—heterochromatin indicates a curtailing of protein synthesis, which is mirrored by a reduction in the organelle population of the cell.

Neutrophilic Stab (band) Cell

—is similar to the mature neutrophil, except for its horseshoe-shaped nucleus. Band cells are frequently found in the circulating blood, and in cases of infection their numbers increase.

Number

—of neutrophils produced in a normal adult is approximately 800,000 per day.

Neutrophil Migration

—occurs in an unusual fashion: the newly formed cells enter the marrow sinusoids by passing through, instead of between, the endothelial cells.

Margination

—occurs in the circulation: a certain percentage of the neutrophils become attached to the endothelial lining of the blood vessel.

Eosinophil and Basophil Formation

—developmental stages of eosinophils and basophils are similar to those described for neutrophils, except that the types of granules formed during the myelocyte stage are specific for each cell type. Also, the morphology of the nucleus in the mature cell resembles that seen in the late band stage.

Monocyte Development
CFU-NM
—a derivative of CFU-S, is the common precursor of monocytes and neutrophils and gives rise to monoblasts.

Monoblasts
—give rise to the promonocyte.

Promonocyte
—is reported to be a large cell (16 to 18 μm diameter) with a somewhat kidney-shaped nucleus located acentrically in a light blue cytoplasm.

—cytoplasm contains numerous azurophilic granules (lysosomes) produced by an extensive Golgi apparatus. Numerous mitochondria and considerable rough endoplasmic reticulum are also present.

Cell Division of Promonocytes
—results in the formation of monocytes, which leave the bone marrow, enter the circulation, and then differentiate into macrophages after they enter the connective tissue.

Number
—of monocytes formed daily in the normal adult is approximately 1×10^{10}.

Platelet Formation
CFU-Meg
—is derived from CFU-S and is not recognizable in histological preparations.

Megakaryoblast
—is a large cell (25 to 40 μm diameter), whose single large nucleus may be indented or lobed but displays a fine chromatin network.

—division of the megakaryoblast occurs endomitotically, in that no daughter cells are formed. Instead the cell becomes huge, and the ploidy of the nucleus may reach 64 N.

—cytoplasm is blue, nongranular, and electron micrographs demonstrate the presence of large mitochondria, numerous polysomes, some rough endoplasmic reticulum, and a fairly well-developed Golgi apparatus.

Megakaryocyte
—an extremely large cell (40 to 100 μm diameter), with a single large polyploid nucleus that is highly lobulated.

—electron micrographs demonstrate that the well-developed Golgi apparatus is actively forming α-granules, lysosomes, and dense bodies. Additionally, this large cell possesses numerous mitochondria and a sizable network of rough endoplasmic reticulum.

—located in the vicinity of sinusoids, where they extend their processes into the sinusoidal lumina.

—processes fragment along some platelet demarcation channels, forming proplatelets (clusters of adhering platelets) that subdivide into single platelets.

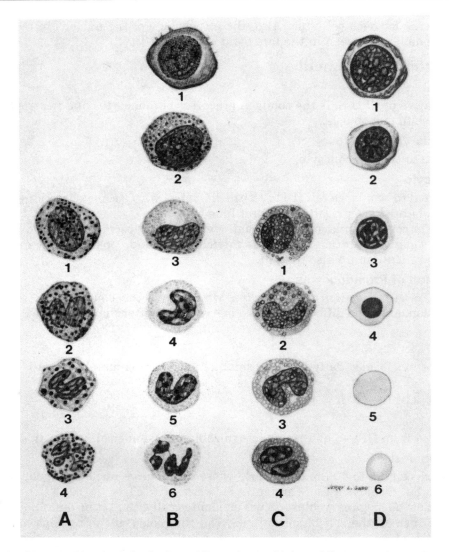

Figure 5.2. Diagram of hemopoiesis. **A1**, basophilic myelocyte; **A2**, basophilic metamyelocyte; **A3**, basophilic stab cell; **A4**, basophil. **B1**, myeloblast; **B2**, promyelocyte; **B3**, neutrophilic myelocyte; **B4**, neutrophilic metamyelocyte; **B5**, neutrophilic stab cell; **B6**, neutrophil. **C1**, eosinophilic myelocyte; **C2**, eosinophilic metamyelocyte; **C3**, eosinophilic stab cell; **C4**, eosinophil. **D1**, proerythroblast; **D2**, basophilic erythroblast; **D3**, polychromatophilic erythroblast; **D4**, orthochromatophilic erythroblast; **D5**, reticulocyte; **D6**, erythrocyte. (From Gartner LP, Hiatt JL: *Atlas of Histology*. Baltimore, Williams & Wilkins, 1987.)

Lymphopoiesis

CFU-Ly

—are derived from THSC (totipotential hemopoietic stem cell) population.

—located in the bone marrow, as well as in circulation as members of the null cell population. They are immunoincompetent cells that give rise to at least two populations of stem cells, CFU-LyT and CFU-LyB [and perhaps CFU-LyNK (natural killer cells)].

CFU-LyB

—pre–B lymphocytes that have not become immunocompetent. These cells replicate rapidly, giving rise to B lymphocytes.

—B lymphocytes become processed to achieve immunocompetence. In birds, processing occurs in an organ called the bursa of Fabricius, hence B lymphocytes; in mammals processing occurs in a bursal equivalent location, probably the bone marrow.

—processed cells migrate to various peripheral organs, such as lymph nodes and spleen, to establish clones of B lymphocytes.

CFU-LyT

—pre–T lymphocytes, i.e., prior to processing. They replicate rapidly, giving rise to T lymphocytes that migrate to the thymus, where they undergo active proliferation to form T lymphocytes.

—T lymphocytes become processed in the thymus. The majority of these newly formed cells are destroyed (in the thymus), while the small percentage that survive migrate to peripheral organs, such as the lymph nodes and spleen, to establish clones of T lymphocytes.

Immunologic Functions

—see Chapter 9 for a discussion of immunologic functions and interactions between classes and subclasses of T and B lymphocytes.

REVIEW TESTS
BLOOD AND HEMOPOIESIS

DIRECTIONS: *One* or *more* of the given completions is/are correct. Choose answer:

    A. if only **1**, **2**, and **3** are correct
    B. if only **1** and **3** are correct
    C. if only **2** and **4** are correct
    D. if only **4** is correct
    E. if **all** are correct

5.1. Serum differs from plasma in that it does not contain the following substance(s)

1. α-globulins
2. γ-globulins
3. albumin
4. fibrinogen

5.2. The following is/are associated with the erythrocyte plasmalemma and is/are responsible for maintaining its biconcave disk shape

1. Hb A_1
2. actin
3. Hb A_2
4. spectrin

5.3. Energy production in mature erythrocytes is accomplished by

1. the glycolytic pathway
2. mitochondria
3. hexose monophosphate shunt
4. citric acid cycle (Krebs cycle)

5.4. Neutrophils

1. possess specific granules that are larger than their azurophilic granules
2. possess specific granules that are smaller than their azurophilic granules
3. form the first line of defense during chronic inflammation
4. avidly phagocytose bacteria

5.5. CFU-S cells give rise to

1. BFU-E
2. CFU-NM
3. CFU-Meg
4. CFU-Ly

5.6. The slow-reacting substance of anaphylaxis is produced by

1. monocytes
2. neutrophils
3. eosinophils
4. basophils

5.7. The term *surface-opening (connecting) tubular system* refers to

1. T lymphocytes
2. B lymphocytes
3. null cells
4. platelets

DIRECTIONS: The following questions or statements refer to the photomicrograph (Fig. 5.3). The letters on the figure are answers to the numbered items appearing below the photomicrograph. For each numbered item select the *one* letter that best corresponds to that item. Each letter may be used once, more than once, or not at all.

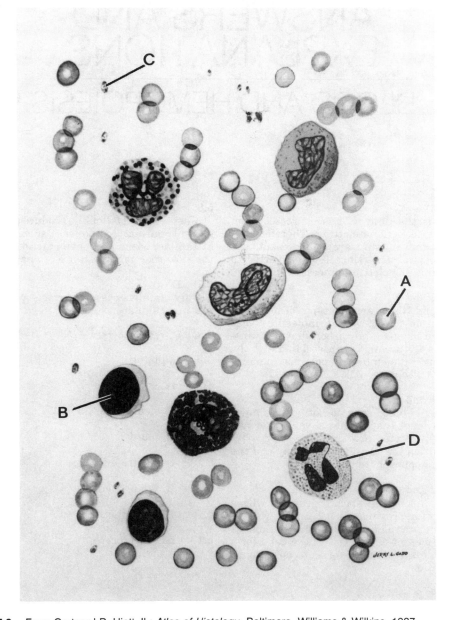

Figure 5.3. From Gartner LP, Hiatt JL: *Atlas of Histology.* Baltimore, Williams & Wilkins, 1987.

5.8. Lymphocyte

5.9. Derived from CFU-Meg

5.10. Derived from BFU-E

5.11. Derived from CFU-NM

5.12. Associated with demarcation channels

5.13. Derived from myeloblasts

5.14. Associated with antibody production

5.15. Possesses specific granules

5.16. Derived from reticulocytes

ANSWERS AND EXPLANATIONS

BLOOD AND HEMOPOIESIS

5.1. D (4)
Serum is the fluid that is expressed from plasma subsequent to clotting. Therefore the globulins and albumin are still present, but fibrinogen is absent (since it is converted to fibrin during the clotting process).

5.2. C (2 and 4)
Hb A_1 and Hb A_2 are two types of hemoglobin, high-molecular-weight molecules that function in oxygen and carbon dioxide transport. Actin and spectrin are associated with the erythrocyte cell membrane and assist in maintaining its biconcave disk shape.

5.3. B (1 and 3)
Mature red blood cells do not possess mitochondria, hence they cannot have a citric acid cycle. Erythrocytes produce their energy requirement via the glycolytic pathway and the hexose monophosphate shunt.

5.4. C (2 and 4)
Neutrophils possess specific granules with a diameter of approximately 0.1 μm, as well as azurophilic granules (lysosomes) with approximate diameters of 0.5 μm. These cells form the first line of defense during acute, not chronic, inflammation.

5.5. A (1, 2, and 3)
Totipotential hemopoietic stem cells (THSC) give rise to CFU-S and CFU-Ly cells. The latter are responsible for the formation of the lymphatic cell lineages, whereas all of the myeloid elements are derived from CFU-S cells.

5.6. D (4)
Mast cells and basophils produce and release several pharmacologic agents, such as heparin, histamine, eosinophil chemotactic factor, and the slow-reacting substance of anaphylaxis.

5.7. D (4)
Only platelets possess surface-opening (connecting) tubular systems.

5.8. B, lymphocyte

5.9. C, platelet

5.10. A, erythrocyte

5.11. D, neutrophil

5.12. C, platelet

5.13. D, neutrophil

5.14. B, lymphocyte

5.15. D, neutrophil

5.16. A, erythrocyte

6
Muscle

Muscle

—one of the four basic tissues.
—classified by its morphology and function.
—striated muscle displays a regular crossbanding pattern and includes skeletal and cardiac muscle.
—smooth muscle lacks crossbanding and is located in the walls of viscera and certain blood vessels.
—contraction of skeletal muscle is voluntary (under conscious control), whereas contraction of both cardiac and smooth muscle is involuntary.

Skeletal Muscle

Organization

Connective Tissue Investments

—associated with muscle at three major levels of organization.
—epimysium surrounds the entire muscle.
—perimysium invests each fascicle.
—endomysium envelopes each fiber (muscle cell).

Fiber Types

Skeletal Muscle

—is heterogeneous in that it is composed of three different types of fibers (cells).
—these fiber types vary in their content of myoglobin pigment, in the number of mitochondria they contain, and in their concentration of various enzymes.

Red Fibers

—contain a large amount of myoglobin pigment, have many mitochondria, and are rich in oxidative enzymes.
—are called slow fibers.
—although easily stimulated, they have a slow conduction rate and are adapted to slow repetitive contractions.
—show weak cytochemical staining for ATPase.

White Fibers

—contain less myoglobin and fewer mitochondria than red fibers.
—are poor in oxidative enzymes but rich in phosphorylases.

—include fast twitch fibers, which have rapid conduction rates and which are adapted to fast, short-lived forces.

—show marked cytochemical staining for ATPase.

Intermediate Fibers

—show features midway between those just described for red and white fibers.

Innervation

—controls the differentiation of fiber types.

—if a red fiber is denervated and replaced by a nerve from a white fiber, the red fiber will change to a white fiber to conform to its new innervation.

Light Microscopy

Skeletal Muscle Fibers (cells)

—are long, multinucleated cells.

—display cross striations that repeat to form a banding pattern.

—in histological sections the A band is anisotropic and appears bright when examined with polarized light, although it is darkly stained with ordinary histological dyes.

—the I band is isotropic and appears dark when examined with polarized light, but it is lightly stained in routine histological preparations.

—the Z line (disk) is a dense area that bisects the I band.

—the H band transects the A band and has a dark M line in its center.

—distance between two successive Z lines is called a sarcomere and is the functional unit of contraction in striated muscle.

Electron Microscopy

Skeletal Muscle Fiber

—is enveloped by a plasma membrane called the sarcolemma.

—has many nuclei lying in a peripheral location just beneath the sarcolemma.

—cytoplasm of the muscle fiber is called the sarcoplasm.

—contains myofibrils extending its entire length.

—crossbanding (an end-to-end chain-like arrangement of sarcomeres) is observed along the myofibrils.

Sarcoplasmic Reticulum

—is a modification of the smooth endoplasmic reticulum.

—surrounds myofilaments and forms a meshwork around each myofibril.

—at the junction of A and I bands, it forms a pair of dilated terminal cisternae, which pass around the myofibrils.

—regulates muscle contraction by sequestering calcium ions (leading to relaxation) or releasing calcium ions (leading to contraction).

Triads

—are a characteristic feature of skeletal muscle.

—located at the A-I junction in mammalian tissue (Fig. 6.1), each triad consists of a narrow transverse tubule (T tubule) between two terminal cisternae of sarcoplasmic reticulum.

—the T tubule is a deep invagination of the sarcolemma (plasma membrane) into the muscle cell.

—between the T tubule and terminal cisternae are regularly spaced densities (junctional feet), which represent areas of low resistance.

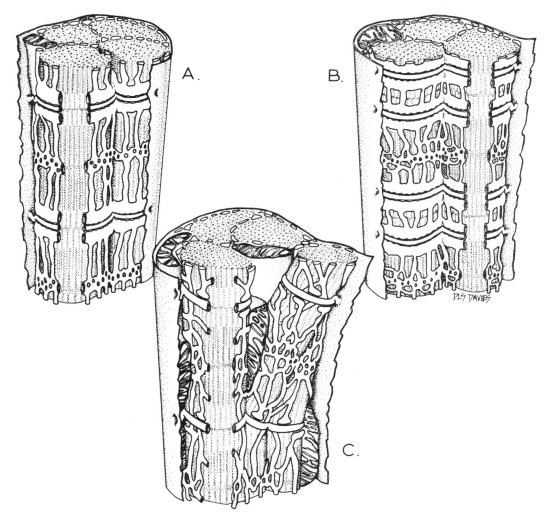

Figure 6.1. Diagrams comparing the organization of T tubules and sarcoplasmic reticula of lower vertebrate (**A**), mammalian skeletal (**B**), and mammalian cardiac muscle fibers (**C**). (From Kelly DE, Wood RL, Enders AC: *Bailey's Textbook of Microscopic Anatomy*, ed 18. Baltimore, Williams & Wilkins, 1984.)

—T tubules rapidly conduct impulses from the exterior of the fiber to deeper regions, where they trigger release of calcium from the terminal cisternae.
—release of calcium into the myofibrils facilitates contraction.

Myofibrils

—consist of longitudinally arranged cylindrical bundles of thick and thin myofilaments.
—lie parallel to the long axis of cell and extend for its entire length.
—display crossbanding characteristic of striated muscle.
—are held in alignment by intermediate filaments composed of the proteins desmin and vimentin.
—are individually surrounded by the sarcoplasmic reticulum.

SKELETAL MUSCLE

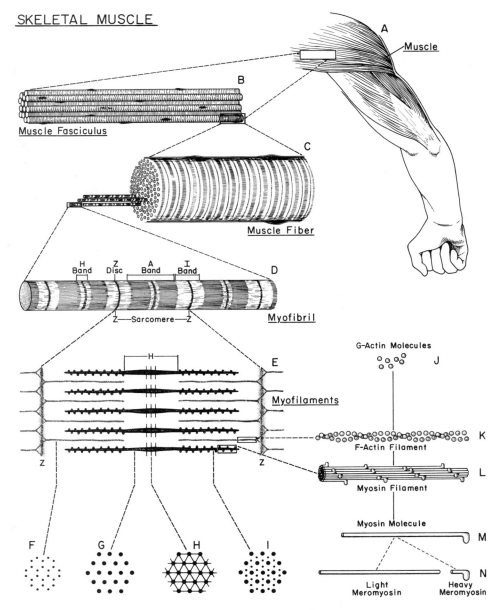

Figure 6.2. Diagram of skeletal muscle and its components as observed in light and electron micrographs. (From Fawcett DW: *Bloom and Fawcett's Textbook of Histology*, ed 11. Philadelphia, WB Saunders, 1986.)

Myofilaments

—are precisely arranged in the myofibril and are responsible for the crossbanding in the sarcomere.

—I band contains only thin filaments, which anchor at the dense Z line.

—A band consists of both thick and thin filaments (making this band birefringent, or anisotropic).

—ratio of thin to thick filaments is 6 to 1.

—M line is formed by cross connections at the midpoints of the thick filaments.

—H band consists of thick filaments only.

Thick Myofilaments

—measure 2 to 3 nm in diameter and 1.5 μm in length.

—are composed of many myosin molecules arranged together to form a rod-like structure.

—each myosin molecule appears similar to a double-headed golf club, with two globular projections, or heads, that possess a specific ATP-binding site.

—ATP hydrolysis occurs at the heads, which is also the location of the actin-binding site.

—myosin is composed of two identical heavy chains and two pairs of light chains.

—heavy chains are enzymatically cleaved to form two fragments, light and heavy meromyosin.

—light meromyosin makes up most of the rod-like portion of the molecule, whereas heavy meromyosin represents the globular head and a small part of the rod.

—cross bridges seen between the thick and thin filaments are formed by the heads of the myosin molecules plus a small part of its rod-like portion.

Thin Myofilaments

—consist primarily of F actin, which is formed by polymerization of G (globular) actin monomers.

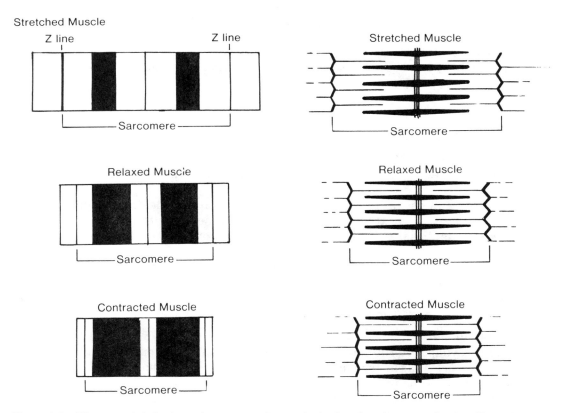

Figure 6.3. Diagrams of skeletal muscle sarcomere in stretched, relaxed, and contracted states. (From Krause WJ, Cutts JH: *Concise Text of Histology*, ed 2. Baltimore, Williams & Wilkins, 1986.)

—measure 5 nm in diameter and 1.0 μm in length.

—each actin filament consists of two such strands in the form of a double helix.

—troponin is distributed along the thin filaments at 40-nm intervals.

—the linear tropomyosin molecule lies within the groove of the actin double helix.

Troponin

—is a complex consisting of three subunits:

—TnC, which binds calcium ions.

—TnT, which binds to tropomyosin.

—TnI, which prevents the interaction between actin and myosin.

Contraction

—is initiated when calcium binds to the TnC unit of troponin.

—this exposes the actin-binding site to the myosin head, which binds to it and splits ATP into ADP, P_i, and energy.

—energy released moves the myosin head, as well as the thin filament bound to it.

—thus the thin filament slides past the thick filament as contraction takes place.

Sliding Filament Hypothesis (of Huxley)

—proposes that the filaments themselves do not change in length but slide past one another to increase the amount of overlap between them.

—sliding action results from repeated "make and break" attachments between the heads of the myosin molecules and neighboring actin filaments.

—result is that the length of the sarcomere is shortened in contraction.

—thin filaments slide to penetrate more deeply into the A band, but the A band remains constant in length.

—I band and H band both decrease in size, as Z lines are drawn closer to the ends of the A bands.

Motor Nerve Ending

Myoneural Junction (motor end plate)

—a specialized region on the skeletal muscle fiber (cell) where a motor nerve terminates.

—as the axon approaches the muscle cell it loses its myelin sheath, but the Schwann cell continues to cover the nonsynaptic surface of the nerve terminal.

—nerve terminal lies in an indentation (primary synaptic cleft) of the skeletal muscle fiber.

—additional invaginations of the sarcolemma lining the primary synaptic cleft form junctional folds (secondary synaptic clefts).

—nerve terminal contains many mitochondria and small vesicles (which are storage sites of the neurotransmitter acetylcholine).

Neural Stimulation

—at the presynaptic terminal stimulates an influx of Ca^{2+} ions, which causes the synaptic vesicles to cluster and release their contents along specialized linear sites (active zones) in the presynaptic membrane.

—acetylcholine released from the vesicles is bound by acetylcholine receptors in the sarcolemma of the muscle cell.

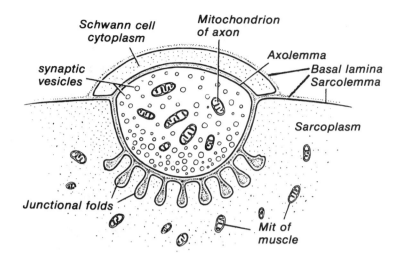

Figure 6.4. Diagram of a myoneural junction as observed in electron micrographs. **Mit of muscle**, mitochondria of muscle. (From Kelly DE, Wood RL, Enders AC: *Bailey's Textbook of Microscopic Anatomy*, ed 18. Baltimore, Williams & Wilkins, 1984.)

—this causes a transient increase in sodium ions, which depolarizes the muscle cell membrane and generates an action potential.

—action potential is propagated over the sarcolemma and into T tubules, activating the release of calcium, which triggers contraction.

—in the basal lamina lining secondary clefts of the motor end plate is acetylcholinesterase, which limits the response to the neurotransmitter by breaking down acetylcholine.

Sensory Nerve Ending

Muscle Spindle (neuromuscular spindle)

—is a sensory organ in skeletal muscle that functions as a stretch receptor.

—muscle spindle receives a large afferent sensory nerve fiber with several types of nerve endings: annulospiral endings (wind around intrafusal fibers); flower spray endings (terminate in clusters); and γ-efferents, or fusimotor endings (form motor endplates near the poles of the spindle).

—appears as an elongated fusiform encapsulated structure that contains several modified striated muscle fibers (intrafusal fibers) and their associated nerve endings.

—intrafusal fibers are of two types:

—nuclear bag fibers have a cluster of nuclei in their nonstriated region that produce a slight expansion in this area.

—thin nuclear chain fibers are the most common; their nuclei are arranged in a row.

Periaxial Space

—a fluid-filled cavity that exists between the connective tissue capsule and the intrafusal fibers.

Figure 6.5. Diagram of a muscle spindle. (From Krause WJ, Cutts JH: *Concise Text of Histology*, ed 2. Baltimore, Williams & Wilkins, 1986.)

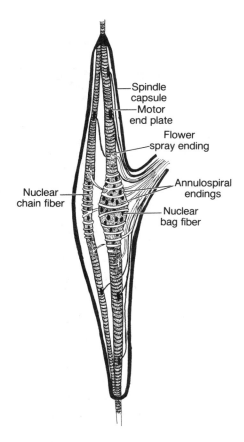

Cardiac Muscle

Characteristics

Striated Muscle Fibers (cells)

—constitute the heart muscle.
—contract spontaneously and display a rhythmic beat.
—are attached end to end by intercalated disks.
—may branch at their ends to form connections with adjacent fibers.
—contain one, or occasionally two, nuclei (located centrally within the cell).
—thick and thin filaments make up poorly defined myofibrils.
—pattern of crossbanding (A, I, and H bands and Z and M lines) is the same as that in skeletal muscle.

T Tubules

—are larger than those of skeletal muscle and are lined by an external (basal) lamina.
—are located at the Z lines in mammalian cardiac muscle (rather than at A-I junctions).

Sarcoplasmic Reticulum

—is poorly developed and contributes to the formation of diads (structures consisting of one T tubule and one profile of sarcoplasmic reticulum).

Mitochondria
—lie parallel to the I bands, and glycogen is common in the cell, especially at either pole of the nucleus.

Atrial Cardiac Muscle Cells
—contain atrial granules in addition to the features just described.
—atrial granules are the source of two polypeptide hormones:

—cardionatrin, a potent natriuretic and diuretic hormone;
—cardiodilatin, a vascular smooth muscle relaxant that facilitates vasodilation.

Intercalated Disks
—are elaborate stepwise junctions forming the end-to-end attachments of adjacent cardiac muscle cells.
—three specializations make up the transverse portion of the intercalated disk: the fascia adherens (an extensive region of adhesion analogous to the zonula adherens), desmosomes, and gap junctions.

Gap Junctions and Desmosomes
—are also common along the longitudinal portion of intercalated disk.
—in heart muscle the transverse portion of the disk substitutes at the Z line.

Purkinje Fibers
—specialized conducting cells of the atrioventricular bundle in the heart.
—are very large modified muscle cells filled with glycogen and containing many mitochondria.
—contain a few myofibrils, which are located peripherally.
—make contact with cardiac muscle cells through gap junctions, desmosomes, and fasciae adherentes (but not through typical intercalated disks).

Smooth Muscle

Characteristics

Smooth Muscle Cells
—are fusiform in shape, with a single, centrally placed nucleus.
—may be arranged in layers, small bundles, or in helical patterns (in arteries).
—are surrounded by a reticular fiber network.
—divide and are important in regeneration.

Nuclei
—are not observed in each cell when smooth muscle is cross-sectioned, since many of them lie outside of the plane of section.
—in the contracted state, if smooth muscle cells are sectioned longitudinally, their nuclei appear accordion-pleated and deeply indented.

Electron Microscopy

Fine Structural Analysis
—of a smooth muscle cell reveals organelles (mitochondria, rough endoplasmic reticulum, Golgi) concentrated near the nucleus.

Organelles
—are involved in the synthesis of type III collagen, elastin, GAGs, glycoproteins, the external lamina, and growth factors.

Cytoplasmic and Peripheral Densities
—in smooth muscle cells are believed to be analogous to Z lines.
—contain α-actinin and function as myofilament attachment sites.
—actin, myosin, and intermediate filaments are also present.
—in nonvascular smooth muscle cells the intermediate filaments are desmin, but in vascular smooth muscle they are vimentin.

Gap Junctions (Nexus)
—between smooth muscle cells facilitate the spread of excitation.

Sarcolemmal Vesicles (caveolae)
—present along the periphery of the cell might function to take up and release calcium ions.

Smooth Endoplasmic Reticulum
—is sparse but closely associated with sarcolemmal vesicles.

Innervation
—of smooth muscle is by sympathetic and parasympathetic nerves of the autonomic nervous system.
—extent of innervation depends on the function and size of the smooth muscle bundle.
—nerve terminals with vesicles containing either acetylcholine (cholinergic nerves) or norepinephrine (noradrenergic nerves) are observed close to the muscle, within the endomysium.

Contraction
—may be initiated in smooth muscle either by nerve impulses, stretching within the muscle itself, or via hormones.
—vascular smooth muscle contraction is usually initiated by a nerve impulse, and there is little spread of conduction from cell to cell.
—visceral smooth muscle contraction is myogenic, and the signal spreads from cell to cell via gap junctions.
—in the uterus, during the terminal stages of pregnancy, smooth muscle cells contract in response to oxytocin.
—elsewhere in the body smooth muscle cells are responsive only to epinephrine.

Myoepithelial Cells

Characteristics
—features are very similar to smooth muscle cells.
—originate from ectoderm in contrast to most smooth muscle cells, which derive from mesoderm.
—are basket-like in shape and have several radiating processes.
—are located between the epithelium and the basal lamina in certain glands (e.g., mammary, submandibular) and ducts.
—contain hemidesmosomes, which attach them to the underlying basal lamina.
—contain actin, myosin, and intermediate (cytokeratin) filaments, as well as cytoplasmic and peripheral densities that serve as attachment sites for them.

—their contraction forces secretory material from the glandular epithelium into the ducts and out of the gland.

Physiological Properties

—of myoepithelial cells vary.

—in the lactating mammary gland they contract in response to oxytocin, and in the lacrimal gland in response to acetylcholine.

REVIEW TESTS

MUSCLE

DIRECTIONS: *One* or *more* of the given completions is/are correct. Choose answer:

- A. if only **1, 2**, and **3** are correct
- B. if only **1** and **3** are correct
- C. if only **2** and **4** are correct
- D. if only **4** is correct
- E. if **all** are correct

6.1. The following is/are *not* under voluntary control:

1. skeletal muscle
2. cardiac muscle
3. the muscle of the tongue
4. smooth muscle

6.2. Endomysium

1. is a connective tissue investment
2. surrounds each fascicle of a muscle
3. surrounds each muscle fiber
4. surrounds the entire muscle

6.3. Z lines

1. are not present in cardiac muscle
2. bisect I bands
3. are absent from smooth muscle
4. function to anchor actin filaments

6.4. Transverse tubules

1. are not present in smooth muscle
2. are extensions of the sarcolemma
3. serve to transmit signals to myofibrils deep within the cell
4. form part of the diads found in cardiac muscle

6.5. Cardiac muscle cells

1. are joined together end to end by intercalated disks
2. contract spontaneously (i.e., without an external stimulus)
3. branch
4. are not well vascularized

6.6. When skeletal muscle contracts

1. the A band decreases in length
2. the I band remains the same length
3. the H band remains the same length
4. the sarcomere decreases in length

DIRECTIONS: Each of the following questions contains five suggested answers. Choose the *one best* response to each question.

6.7. All of the following statements are true of mature skeletal muscle *except*

A. the cells are multinucleated
B. a sarcomere is the distance between two successive Z lines
C. the nuclei are centrally located
D. myofibrils display the characteristic crossbanding pattern
E. actin, myosin, tropomyosin, and troponin are present

6.8. A triad in mammalian skeletal muscle

A. is located at the Z line
B. consists of two terminal cisternae separated by a slender T tubule
C. cannot be observed in electron micrographs
D. is characterized by a T tubule that sequesters calcium
E. consists of two T tubules separated by a narrow central terminal cisterna

6.9. Smooth muscle
A. can be induced to contract by an act of the will
B. does not contain gap junctions
C. does not contain intermediate filaments
D. has cells with centrally located nuclei
E. has cells that contain few, if any, sarcolemmal vesicles

6.10. All of the following statements are true of sarcoplasmic reticulum *except*
A. it is associated with each myofibril in a skeletal muscle cell
B. it binds calcium ions
C. it forms part of the diad in cardiac muscle
D. it communicates with the extracellular space at the surface of the sarcolemma
E. it releases calcium after receiving a signal for contraction

---

DIRECTIONS: The following statements or items refer to the light and electron micrographs (Figures 6.6 and 6.7). Select the *one* lettered structure that is most closely associated with each of the following descriptive phrases or items. Each letter may be used once, more than once, or not at all.

For questions **6.11** and **6.12**, see Figure 6.6.

6.11. Intercalated disk

6.12. Myofibrils

For questions **6.13** through **6.15**, see Figure 6.7.

6.13. Z line

6.14. Band where thin filaments only are present

6.15. Band where thick filaments only are present

Figure 6.6. From Gartner LP, Hiatt JL: *Atlas of Histology.* Baltimore, Williams & Wilkins, 1987.

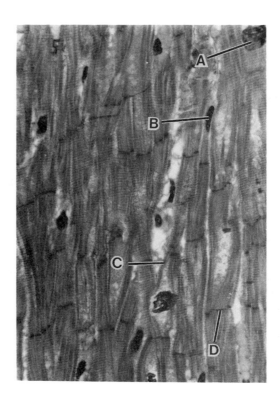

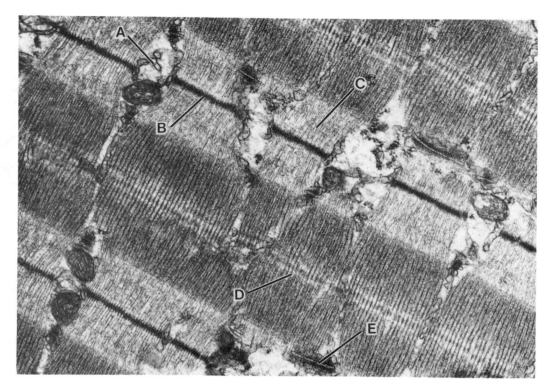

Figure 6.7. From Gartner LP, Hiatt JL: *Atlas of Histology*. Baltimore, Williams & Wilkins, 1987.

ANSWERS AND EXPLANATIONS

MUSCLE

6.1. C (2 and 4)
Skeletal muscle, including that of the tongue, is subject to voluntary control. In contrast, cardiac and smooth muscle are regulated by the autonomic nervous system and are not subject to voluntary control.

6.2. B (1and 3)
Endomysium consists of reticular and collagen fibers and is a connective tissue investment of each muscle fiber (cell). The individual fascicles in a muscle are invested by perimysium, and the entire muscle is surrounded by epimysium.

6.3. C (2 and 4)
Z lines are a characteristic feature of skeletal and cardiac muscle. They transect I bands and function to anchor thin actin filaments. Since smooth muscle lacks typical "striations," Z lines are not present.

6.4. E (all are correct)
Transverse tubules are present within skeletal and cardiac muscle and are formed by a deep invagination of the plasmalemma. Each transverse tubule functions to carry the depolarization signal into the depths of the cell, where it triggers the mechanism responsible for enabling the myofibrils to undergo contraction. Transverse tubules are absent from smooth muscle.

6.5. A (1, 2, and 3)
Cardiac muscle cells are inherently contractile and do so in a rhythmic manner. They branch and are joined together end to end by a unique junctional specialization called the intercalated disk. Cardiac muscle is richly vascularized.

6.6. D (4)
During contraction both the thick and thin filaments of skeletal muscle retain their original length but slide in relationship to one another, thus increasing the amount of overlap between the filaments. Therefore, during contraction the A band retains the same dimension, but the I and H bands decrease in size (as the thin filaments penetrate deeply into and beyond the A band).

6.7. C
In mature skeletal muscle the nuclei have a peripheral location just deep to the sarcolemma.

6.8. B
A triad in skeletal muscle is composed of three structures, the T tubule and the two terminal cisternae that flank it. In mammalian muscle, triads are located at the A-I junctions and can only be observed in electron micrographs. The function of the T tubule is to conduct impulses to myofibrils deep within the cell.

6.9. D
Nuclei are centrally located in smooth muscle cells. The muscle is involuntary and contains gap junctions, intermediate filaments, and many sarcolemmal vesicles.

6.10. D
The sarcoplasmic reticulum does not communicate with the extracellular space at the surface of the sarcolemma, but the T tubule does. All of the other statements about the sarcoplasmic reticulum are true.

For questions **6.11** and **6.12**, refer to Figure 6.6.

6.11. D

6.12. C

For questions **6.13** through **6.15**, refer to Figure 6.7.

6.13. B

6.14. C

6.15 D

7

Nervous Tissue

Components and Divisions of the Nervous Tissue

Neurons
—the specialized cells of the nervous system.
—have the capacity to conduct an impulse to higher centers for processing, and from these centers a response is initiated.

Glial Cells
—are also part of the nervous system, and they support, nurture, and protect the neurons.

Anatomical Divisions
—central nervous system (CNS) and peripheral nervous system (PNS).
—CNS is represented by the brain and spinal cord.
—PNS includes the nerves and their associated ganglia.

Functional Divisions
—sensory and motor components.
—sensory component collects information from the internal and external environment and transmits it to centers in the CNS for processing and analysis.
—motor component delivers impulses from the CNS to various structures of the body that effect organized and coordinated responses: somatic (voluntary) system controls skeletal muscle; autonomic (involuntary) system, composed of sympathetic and parasympathetic components, controls smooth muscle, cardiac muscle, and glands.

Development

Nervous System
—develops from the neuroepithelium comprising the early neural plate, just before the neural groove folds to form the neural tube.
—neural crest cells stream off edges of the neural groove folds and migrate throughout the body to form ganglia, the adrenal medulla, etc.
—cranial end of the neural tube enlarges to form the brain, and the remaining portion forms the spinal cord.

Cells

Neurons

—consist of a cell body (soma, perikaryon) and its processes, which include the dendrites, and an axon.

—dendrites conduct information toward the soma.

—axons conduct information away from it.

—largest and smallest cells of the body, ranging from 4 to 5 μm (cells of the cerebellum) up to 150 μm in diameter.

Morphological Classification of Neurons

—unipolar neurons possess an axon and only one dendrite.

—bipolar neurons possess a single axon and a single dendrite.

—multipolar neurons possess an axon and more than one dendrite.

—pseudounipolar neurons possess what appears to be a single process extending from the soma, which subsequently branches into an axon and a dendrite. These originate embryologically as a bipolar cell, but the axon and dendrite fuse into a single process.

Functional Classification

—of neurons includes sensory, motor, and interneurons.

—sensory neurons receive stimuli from the environment.

—interneurons act as connectors of neurons in a chain or sequence.

—motor neurons conduct impulses to other neurons, muscles, or glands.

Soma (cell body)

—region of the neuron containing the nucleus and most of the organelles of the cell.

—nucleus is large, spherical, and pale-staining, with finely dispersed chromatin and a large nucleolus. The nucleus is centrally located in the soma of most neurons; in

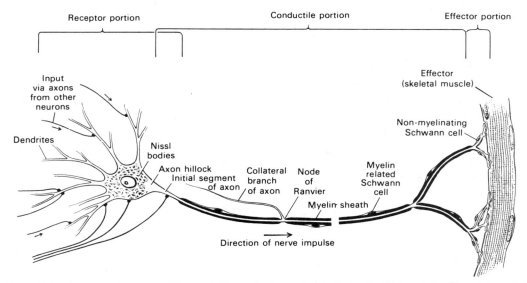

Figure 7.1. Diagram of a neuron. The gap in its conducting portion indicates that its length has been interrupted. (From Kelly DE, Wood RL, Enders AC: *Bailey's Textbook of Microscopic Anatomy*, ed 18. Baltimore, Williams & Wilkins, 1984.)

females the nucleus often displays a Barr body (sex chromatin) located at various sites in the nucleoplasm.

—Nissl bodies (most abundant in large motor nerve cells) are rosettes of polysomes and rough endoplasmic reticulum, observed as basophilic clumps in light microscopy.

—Golgi apparatus, located near the nucleus, is composed of smooth cisternae or saccules, vacuoles, and adjacent small vesicles.

—mitochondria are scattered through the soma cytoplasm but are especially abundant near the axon terminals.

—neurofilaments (10 nm intermediate filaments) are profuse in the cell and run throughout the cytoplasm. The neurofibrils seen by light microscopy are fixation artifacts and represent aggregated neurofilaments.

—microtubules (24 nm diameter) are also present in the cytoplasm of the nerve cell body.

—inclusions in neurons vary, depending on the location of the cells: melanin pigment is observed in certain neurons located in the CNS and in spinal and sympathetic ganglia; lipofuscin is present in certain neurons, becoming more abundant with age; lipid droplets are occasionally present.

Dendrites

—receive information and transmit it toward the cell body. Most dendrite terminals (with the exception of those in bipolar neurons) are arborized, permitting them to receive information simultaneously from a multitude of axons at the sites of synaptic contact.

—cytoplasm is similar in composition to that of the cell body, except that it lacks a Golgi apparatus.

Axons

—vary in diameter and length (some are as long as 100 cm).

—originate from the axon hillock, a specialized region of the soma devoid of rough endoplasmic reticulum and ribosomes.

—collaterals occasionally branch at right angles from the trunk of an axon.

—axoplasm (cytoplasm) is surrounded by the axolemma (plasma membrane) and possesses only a few organelles, since it has low synthetic activity.

Synapse

—site where information is transferred between a neuron and another cell. Various types of synapses exist.

—axodendritic synapse: site of contact between an axon and a dendrite.
—axosomatic synapse: site of contact between an axon and a nerve cell body.
—axoaxonic synapse: site of contact between axons.
—dendodendritic synapse: site of contact between dendrites.

Terminals

—may vary morphologically at synaptic sites and be of several varieties.
—bouton terminaux: a singular basket-shaped terminal.
—boutons en passage: swellings along the terminal where several synapses are present.

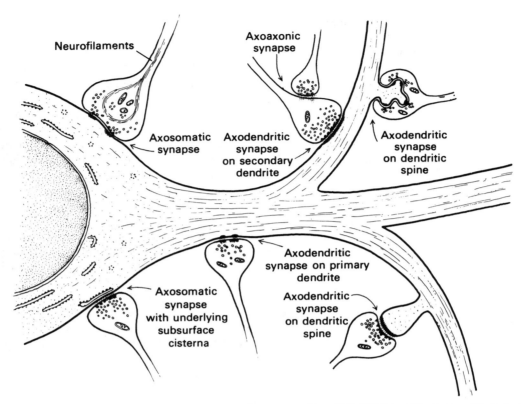

Figure 7.2. Diagram illustrating the various types of synapses. (From Kelly DE, Wood RL, Enders AC: *Bailey's Textbook of Microscopic Anatomy*, ed 18. Baltimore, Williams & Wilkins, 1984.)

Chemical Synapses
—involve the transmission of information from one cell to the next by the release of neurotransmitter substances (e.g., acetylcholine, GABA, norepinephrine).
—cells display densities at the plasmalemma and filaments extend into these dense areas.
—enzymes located in the synaptic cleft between the pre- and postsynaptic membranes cleave and inactivate excess neurotransmitter.

Presynaptic Membrane
—the thickened plasma membrane of the nerve cell discharging the impulse. Calcium gates that help facilitate the fusion of synaptic vesicles with the presynaptic membrane are located at this region.

Postsynaptic Membrane
—the thickened plasma membrane of the nerve cell receiving the impulse.

Synaptic Cleft
—a narrow space (20 to 30 nm width) between the pre- and postsynaptic membranes. Fine filaments and occasionally dense material are found occupying this region.

Synaptic Vesicles
—small membrane-bounded structures (40 to 60 nm diameter) located near the pre-synaptic membrane in the cytoplasm of the discharging cell.
—contain neurotransmitter substance. They are responsible for transmission of the impulse. The synaptic vesicles discharge the neurotransmitter into the synaptic gap via exocytosis.
—vesicle membrane thus becomes incorporated into the presynaptic membrane. It then undergoes endocytosis (combining with clathrin to form coated vesicles) and is recycled to form new vesicles.
—released neurotransmitter crosses the synaptic cleft and binds to receptors on the postsynaptic membrane, thus propagating the impulse.

Electrical Synapses
—occur where ions are passed from neuron to neuron to generate an action potential.
—appear as gap junctions and have plaque-like specializations associated with their plasma membranes.

Neuroglia
—cells located in the CNS that function to support neurons. They outnumber neurons by approximately 10 to 1 and are revealed in histological sections only with special gold and silver stains.
—types: astrocytes, oligodendrocytes, microglia, and ependymal cells.

Astrocytes
—the largest neuroglial cells. They have many processes, the terminals of which are enlarged to form vascular feet and ensheathe blood vessels.
—are located beneath the pia of the brain and spinal cord.
—electron micrographs reveal an electron-lucent, nearly organelle-free cytoplasm containing many microfibrils.
—protoplasmic astrocytes: reside in gray matter of the CNS.
—fibrous astrocytes: are located in white matter.
—function: provide most of the supporting elements for the nervous system.
—assist in the maintenance of electrolyte balance in the CNS.
—vascular feet transport bloodborne nutrients to neurons.

Oligodendrocytes
—small glial cells located in the CNS that have only a few short processes.
—live symbiotically with neurons, in that each is affected by the metabolic activities of the other and neurons are not able to survive without oligodendrocytes.
—electron micrographs display a small, round, condensed nucleus and an electron-dense cytoplasm that contains ribosomes, microtubules, and mitochondria.
—function to produce myelin in the CNS; each cell can myelinate several axons.
—form a protective barrier around the neurons, serving to insulate them.

Microglia
—small cells in the CNS having short processes that contain many small branches.
—contain a very condensed, elongated nucleus.
—are derived from monocytes of the bone marrow and are phagocytic.

Ependymal Cells
—form the epithelium that lines the neural tube and ventricles of the brain.
—during development, ependymal cell processes extend between neural elements as far as the pia mater and form a supporting framework for the system.

Nerve Fibers

Axons
—of neurons enveloped in myelin sheaths produced by Schwann cells (in the PNS) or by oligodendrocytes (in the CNS) are referred to as myelinated axons. Axons not enveloped by myelin are said to be unmyelinated.
—as axon diameter increases, myelin sheath thickness also usually increases.
—unmyelinated axons are not enveloped by myelin and are usually small.

Myelin
—a lipoprotein organized into a sheath that is formed by several layers of plasma membrane of oligodendrocytes or Schwann cells wrapping around the axon.
—histological processing removes myelin, but methods using osmium tetroxide preserve it.
—electron micrographs display major dense lines and intraperiod lines: major dense lines represent fusions between the cytoplasmic surfaces of Schwann cell (or oligodendroglia) plasmalemmae; intraperiod lines represent close contact between extracellular surfaces of Schwann cell (or oligodendroglia) plasma membranes.
—myelin sheath does not uniformly cover the axon but covers it in a fashion resembling a string of beads, where the beads represent the myelin.

Node of Ranvier
—represents regions of discontinuities between adjacent Schwann cells (or oligodendroglia). The axolemma at the node displays a unique electron density that is characteristic of this area.

Internode
—represents the distance between nodes. It varies in dimension, depending on the size of the Schwann cell (or oligodendroglia), from 0.08 to 1 mm.
—displays oblique discontinuities called clefts or incisures of Schmidt-Lanterman.

Unmyelinated Fibers
—axons that do not possess myelin sheaths but are ensheathed by oligodendroglia (in the CNS) or Schwann cells (in the PNS).

Nerves
—bundles of individual nerve fibers wrapped in connective tissue (fascial) sheaths.

Epineurium
—the outer layer of dense connective tissue surrounding bundles of nerve fibers and extending into the spaces between them.

Perineurium
—the connective tissue investment around individual nerve fascicles.
—consists of layers of epithelioid cells that are joined by tight junctions.
—functions as a barrier to most macromolecules.

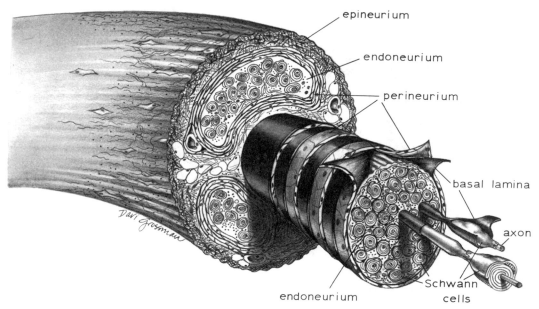

Figure 7.3. Diagram of the various connective tissue sheaths of a peripheral nerve. (From Kelly DE, Wood RL, Enders AC: *Bailey's Textbook of Microscopic Anatomy*, ed 18. Baltimore, Williams & Wilkins, 1984.)

Endoneurium

—a thin layer of connective tissue investing individual nerve fibers.

Sensory Nerves

—afferent fibers that carry only sensory information from the internal and external environment to the CNS.

Motor Nerves

—efferent fibers that only carry impulses from the CNS to effector organs.

Mixed Nerves

—the most common and contain both sensory and motor fibers.

Autonomic Nervous System

—a motor system that controls and regulates smooth muscle, cardiac muscle, and glands.
—establishes and maintains homeostasis with regard to visceral function.
—its neurons originate in the CNS.
—its preganglionic fibers (axons) extend to a ganglion (located in the PNS), where they synapse with a second neuron in the chain, called a postganglionic soma.
—its postganglionic fiber (axon) leaves the ganglion to terminate in the effector organ (smooth muscle, cardiac muscle, gland).
—is subdivided anatomically and functionally into the sympathetic and the parasympathetic nervous systems.

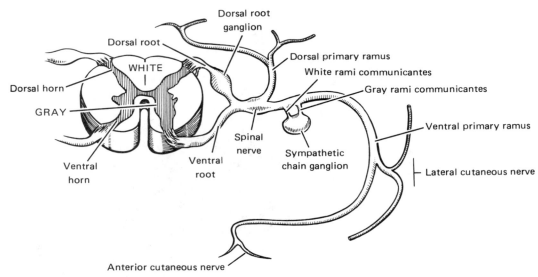

Figure 7.4. Diagram of a typical thoracic spinal cord segment and typical spinal nerve. (From Hiatt JL, Gartner LP: *Textbook of Head and Neck Anatomy*, ed 2. Baltimore, Williams & Wilkins, 1987.)

Sympathetic System (thoracolumbar outflow)

—cell bodies of preganglionic fibers in this system are located in the thoracic and first two lumbar spinal cord segments.

Preganglionic Axons

—leave the spinal cord via the ventral root of a spinal nerve and enter one of the ganglia of the sympathetic system, where they synapse on postganglionic cell bodies.

—acetylcholine is the neurotransmitter of preganglionic synapses.

Postganglionic Axons

—leave the ganglion to find their way to the effector organ (smooth muscle, cardiac muscle, glands).

—norepinephrine is the neurotransmitter of postganglionic synapses.

Parasympathetic System (craniosacral outflow)

—cell bodies of preganglionic fibers are located in certain cranial nerve nuclei within the brain and some segments of the sacral spinal cord.

—axons of preganglionic fibers leave the brain or spinal cord and enter parasympathetic ganglia, where they synapse with postganglionic fibers that are distributed to the effector organs (smooth muscle, cardiac muscle, glands).

Parasympathetic Ganglia

—in the head are located some distance away from the effector organs; postganglionic fibers are distributed by cranial nerves.

—visceral ganglia in the remainder of the body are located close to the effector organs (often within their walls); postganglionic fibers are very short.

—acetylcholine is the neurotransmitter for both pre- and postganglionic synapses in the parasympathetic nervous system.

Distribution
—generally in organs where the sympathetic system functions to stimulate, the parasympathetic system functions to inhibit, and vice versa.

Function
—stimulates secretion (secretomotor) and acts in vasoconstriction.

Histophysiology
—neurons conduct nerve impulses from one neuron to another and/or to effector organs.
—potassium concentration inside a neuron is about 20 times greater than it is in the extracellular fluid.
—sodium concentration is about 10 times greater extracellularly than intracellularly.
—potassium diffuses outward, setting up a positive charge outside the cell membrane that is offset by negative charges within the cell (produced by anionic particles to which the membrane is impermeable).

Resting Membrane Potential
—occurs when a balance is reached between the concentration gradient and the diffusion force, such that there are no net movements of potassium ions across the membrane.
—extracellular fluid is considered to be at ground potential (0 V), whereas the interior of the cell is about 40 to 100 mV negative, compared with the outside.

Sodium Pump
—maintains concentration differences by using energy from ATP to transport (active transport) internal sodium in exchange for external potassium.

Voltage-Gated Channels
—exist in plasma membranes of neurons and muscle cells whose membrane proteins are ion-selective.
—channels may be open, closed, or inactivated.

Action Potential
—excitatory synaptic input on the postsynaptic cell depolarizes a portion of the plasma membrane, and as the membrane potential is depressed a critical threshold is reached.
—threshold opens sodium membrane channels, permitting sodium ions to enter the cell, which produces further membrane depolarization, reversing the membrane potential at this site.
—sodium channels become inactivated for 1 to 2 ms (refractory period), and at the same time potassium channels open (for longer periods of time), causing the membrane potential to return to its normal level or to a hyperpolarized state.
—channels return to their original states after the refractory period, resetting the membrane for a response to another stimulus. This series of events makes up an action potential.
—action potentials are developed from this series of events, and axons are able to generate them up to 1000 times per second.

Antidromic Spread
—a diffusion of sodium ions, toward the cell body and away from the activated site, that has no effect on depolarization since the sodium channels are inactivated.

Orthodromic Spread

—a diffusion of sodium ions, toward the synaptic end of the axon, that gives rise to a new action potential that is propagated down the axon.

Saltatory Conduction

—the rapid conduction of an action potential that occurs from node to node in a myelinated fiber.

—nodes of Ranvier are unmyelinated areas of a myelinated axon that are directly exposed to the external environment and thus able to generate action potentials very rapidly.

—transmission in unmyelinated fibers is much slower.

Types of Nerve Fibers

—affect impulse transmission rates.

—type A fibers are large, myelinated, have long internodes, and conduct impulses at high rates of speed (15 to 100 m/s).

—type B fibers have moderate diameters, a thinner layer of myelin, and conduct impulses at a moderate velocity (3 to 14 m/s).

—type C fibers are thin, unmyelinated, and have a relatively slow impulse velocity (0.5 to 2 m/s).

Neurotransmitters

—liberated at the synapse, change plasma membrane permeability and facilitate the propagation of an impulse.

—acetylcholine is the neurotransmitter at parasympathetic and preganglionic sympathetic synapses.

—norepinephrine is the neurotransmitter at postganglionic sympathetic synapses.

—additional neurotransmitters also exist, such as γ-aminobutyric acid (GABA), glutamic acid, dopamine, serotonin, and glycine.

—brain-produced peptide neurotransmitters are inhibitors of pain and include endorphins and enkephalins.

Axonal Transport

—occurs in neurons. Some substances are transported at high speeds, others at intermediate, and still others at lower velocities.

—anterograde transport is transport away from the soma.

—retrograde transport is transport toward the soma.

Trophic Function

—the nervous system exhibits a trophic function on the organs it innervates. Thus denervating a muscle or a gland leads to its atrophy, whereas reinnervation restores its structure and function.

Degeneration and Regeneration

Neurons

—are unable to divide, but glial cells can divide and they fill in areas left by dead neurons.

—are able to regenerate lost or injured processes, provided the perikaryon has not been destroyed.

Degeneration

—occurs when a neuron is injured and its distal process is no longer in contact with the perikaryon.

—distal process degenerates, and its remnants are removed by macrophages.

—proximal portion still in contact with the perikaryon may regenerate.

Injured Axons

—induce changes in the perikaryon, including chromatolysis (dissolution of Nissl substance and a loss of cytoplasmic basophilia), increase in the volume of the perikaryon, and movement of its nucleus to a peripheral position.

—distal end of the proximal portion of the axon (next to the injury) degenerates.

—regeneration follows after remnants are removed and Schwann cells organize into columns to guide the sprouting axon.

Ganglia

—are encapsulated aggregations of nerve cell bodies outside the CNS. Several categories of ganglia exist.

Autonomic Ganglia

—are associated with autonomic nerves. They contain the cell bodies of postganglionic neurons that are usually multipolar.

—small satellite cells often surround the nerve cell bodies.

Intramural Ganglia

—are included within the autonomic category. They are part of the parasympathetic system and contain nerve cell bodies located in the walls of viscera.

Meissner's and Auerbach's Plexuses

—contain intramural ganglia.

Craniospinal Ganglia

—are sensory ganglia associated with most cranial nerves and the dorsal roots of spinal nerves (dorsal root ganglia).

—contain pseudounipolar neurons whose function is to transmit sensory information into the CNS from sensory receptors.

Gray and White Matter

—both gray and white matter are contained in the CNS.

Gray Matter

—contains nerve cell bodies, many unmyelinated fibers, and some myelinated fibers, along with glial cells.

White Matter

—contains mostly myelinated nerve fibers, but unmyelinated fibers and glial cells are also present.

Spinal Cord Gray Matter

—appears in the shape of an H, and a small canal occupies the center of the crossbar in the H.

—central canal is lined by ependymal cells and represents the lumen of the embryonic neural tube.

—upper bars of the H are dorsal horns, which receive sensory fibers from the dorsal
   root ganglia.
—lower bars of the H represent and contain large multipolar motor neurons.

Brain Gray Matter (cerebrum and cerebellum)
—is located at the periphery and white matter is deep to it.

Meninges

Dura Mater
—the outermost dense fibrous connective tissue covering of the brain and spinal cord.
   Although it is continuous with the periosteum of the skull, an epidural space separates it from the periosteum of the vertebrae.
—simple squamous cells line its internal surface in the brain and both sides of it in
   the spinal cord.

Arachnoid
—the middle layer of the meninges, lying between the dura mater and the pia mater.
—is covered on either side by a simple squamous epithelium and has trabeculae that
   form a loose network between it and the pia.
—trabeculae extend into the subarachnoid space that is filled with cerebrospinal fluid.

Arachnoid Villi
—are specialized regions of the arachnoid that protrude through the dura to a venous
   space and return cerebrospinal fluid into the venus sinuses.

Pia Mater
—the innermost layer of the meninges lying over the brain and spinal cord. It contains
   many blood vessels, and squamous cells cover its surface.
—thin layer of glial elements lies between the pia and the nervous tissue.

Choroid Plexus
—consists of folds of the pia mater that extend into the third, fourth, and lateral
   ventricles of the brain.
—is composed of a core of connective tissue covered by a simple cuboidal epithelium
   having many microvilli.
—connective tissue is vascular and contains many fenestrated capillaries, and the
   cerebrospinal fluid is a product of the epithelial layer.
—secretes cerebrospinal fluid.

Cerebrospinal Fluid
—elaborated by the choroid plexus, bathes and nourishes the brain and spinal cord,
   filling the ventricles, spinal canal, subarachnoid space, and perivascular space.
—surrounds the entire CNS and protects it by acting as a cushion.
—contains little protein but is rich in sodium, potassium, and chloride. The fluid is
   continuously produced by the choroid plexus and is reabsorbed by the arachnoid
   villi that transport it into the superior sagittal sinus.
—blockage in reabsorption leads to hydrocephalus.

Cerebral Cortex
—Cerebral Cortex: is responsible for several diverse functions, such as memory, learn-
   ing, association and analysis of information, initiating motor responses, and inte-
   gration of incoming data.

—is composed of six layers; molecular layer, external granular layer, external pyramidal layer, internal granular layer, internal pyramidal layer, and the deepest layer, the multiform layer.

—Molecular layer: houses only a few soma, and numerous neuroglia.

—External granular layer: is composed of granule cells and neuroglia.

—External pyramidal layer: consists of pyramidal cells, some granule cells, and neuroglia.

—Internal granular layer: is a relatively narrow band that is composed of small and large granule cells and neuroglia.

—Internal pyramidal layer: houses medium and large pyramidal cells and neuroglia.

—Multiform layer: contains cells of various shapes, many of which are fusiform. This layer also houses Martinotti cells and neuroglia.

Cerebellar Cortex

—Cerebellar cortex: functions in maintenance of balance, equilibrium, muscle tone, and coordination of skeletal muscle activity.

—is composed of three layers; the molecular layer, the layer of Purkinje cells, and the deepest layer, the granular layer.

—Molecular layer: contains unmyelinated fibers from the granular layer, the superficially located stellate cells, and basket cells.

—Purkinje cell layer: is composed of the huge, Purkinje cells, characteristic of the cerebellar cortex.

—Purkinje cells: are located in a single layer, possess a flask shaped soma and a centrally placed nucleus.

—its myelinated axon enters the granular layer, whereas its dendrites arborize, in a single plane, in the molecular layer. It is estimated that each Purkinje cell may receive several hundred thousands of excitatory and inhibitory impulses which they must sort and integrate.

—Granular layer: is composed of closely packed small granule cells and interspersed among them are regions apparently devoid of cells, known as cerebellar islands (glomeruli).

—Cerebellar islands: are areas where synapses occur between axons entering the cerebellum from the outside and dendrites of granule cells.

REVIEW TESTS
NERVOUS TISSUE

DIRECTIONS: *One* or *more* of the given completions or answers is/are correct. Choose answer:

    A. if only **1, 2,** and **3** are correct
    B. if only **1** and **3** are correct
    C. if only **2** and **4** are correct
    D. if only **4** is correct
    E. if **all** are correct

7.1. Neural crest cells give rise to
1. dorsal root ganglia
2. adrenal medulla
3. sympathetic ganglia
4. all peripheral nerves

7.2. Myelination is produced by
1. astrocytes
2. oligodendrocytes
3. neural crest cells
4. Schwann cells

7.3. During chromatolysis
1. the nucleus becomes smaller
2. the perikaryon shrinks
3. Nissl body is increased
4. the nucleus becomes eccentric in the perikaryon

7.4. Neurons possess
1. neurotubules
2. neurofilaments
3. Nissl body
4. mitochondria

7.5. Cholinergic synapses occur in
1. preganglionic parasympathetic synapses
2. preganglionic sympathetic synapses
3. postganglionic parasympathetic synapses
4. postganglionic sympathetic synapses

7.6. Neuroglial cells include
1. astrocytes
2. ependymal cells
3. microglia
4. neurons

7.7 Nissl bodies are composed of
1. synaptic vesicles
2. free ribosomes
3. lipoprotein
4. rough endoplasmic reticulum

7.8. Synaptic vesicles
1. contain neurotransmitters
2. enter the synaptic gap
3. become incorporated in the presynaptic membrane after emptying contents
4. become incorporated in the postsynaptic membrane

DIRECTIONS: Each of the following questions contains four suggested answers. Choose the *one best* response to each question.

7.9. The axon hillock
A. contains rough endoplasmic reticulum
B. contains ribosomes
C. contains microtubules arranged in bundles
D. contains all of the above

7.10. The perineurium
A. is a fascial layer surrounding bundles of nerve fibers
B. is a cellular layer surrounding individual bundles of nerves
C. is a thin layer of connective tissue covering individual nerves
D. is composed of mostly reticular fibers

7.11. Cell bodies of preganglionic sympathetic neurons
A. are housed in the brain
B. are housed in the thoracic spinal cord
C. are found throughout the CNS
D. are found in sympathetic ganglia only

7.12. Neurotransmitters include
A. acetylcholine
B. norepinephrine
C. enkephalins
D. all of the above

DIRECTIONS: The following questions or statements refer to the photomicrograph (Fig. 7.5). The letters on the figure are answers to the numbered items appearing below the photomicrograph. For each numbered item, select the *one* letter that *best* corresponds to that item. Each letter may be used once, more than once, or not at all.

Figure 7.5. From Gartner LP, Hiatt JL: *Atlas of Histology*. Baltimore, Williams & Wilkins, 1987.

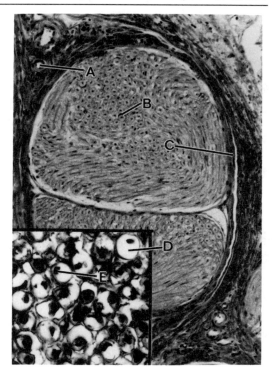

7.13. Perineurium

7.14. Axon

7.15. Myelin

ANSWERS AND EXPLANATIONS

NERVOUS TISSUE

7.1. A (1, 2, and 3)
The neural crest cells give rise to the dorsal root ganglia, adrenal medulla, and the autonomic ganglia. Peripheral nerves do not derive from neural crest.

7.2. C (2 and 4)
Oligodendrocytes produce the myelin in the CNS, whereas Schwann cells produce myelin in the peripheral nerves. Astrocytes and neural crest cells do not produce myelin.

7.3. D (4)
During chromatolysis the nucleus becomes eccentric in the perikaryon and Nissl body is decreased.

7.4. E (1, 2, 3, and 4)
Neurons possess neurotubules, neurofilaments, Nissl body, and mitochondria.

7.5. A (1, 2, and 3)
Cholinergic synapses occur in pre- and postganglionic parasympathetic synapses and in preganglionic sympathetic synapses. Norepinephrine is the neurotransmitter of the postganglionic sympathetic synapse.

7.6. A (1, 2, and 3)
Astrocytes, ependymal cells, and microglia are all neuroglial cells. The neuron is the functional cell of the nervous system.

7.7. C (2 and 4)
Nissl body is a special configuration of ribosomes and rough endoplasmic reticulum in a neuron cell body.

7.8. B (1 and 3)
Synaptic vesicles contain neurotransmitters and become incorporated into the presynaptic membrane after the neurotransmitter has been released into the synaptic gap.

7.9. C
The axon hillock contains microtubules arranged in bundles.

7.10. B
The cellular layer that surrounds individual bundles of nerves is the perineurium. It also serves as a barrier for macromolecules.

7.11. B
Cell bodies of sympathetic neurons are housed in the thoracic spinal cord and first two segments of the lumbar spinal cord. Additionally the postganglionic cell bodies are housed in sympathetic ganglia. They are not found in the brain or throughout the entire CNS.

7.12. D
There are several groups of neurotransmitters. Acetylcholine, norepinephrine, and enkephalins are all neurotransmitters.

7.13. Perineurium (C)

7.14. Axon (E)

7.15. Myelin (D)

8

Circulatory System

Circulatory System

—includes the vascular systems that carry both blood and lymph.

Blood Vascular System
—includes the heart (a four-chambered pump) and a system of vessels: the arteries, veins, and capillaries.
—arteries convey blood from the heart to the tissues of the body.
—veins return blood from the tissues back to the heart.
—capillaries are interposed between the arteries and veins and provide oxygen and nutrients to the surrounding tissues in exchange for carbon dioxide and waste materials.

Lymphatic System
—returns tissue fluids to the bloodstream.
—begins as blind-ended vessels in the tissues, called lymphatic capillaries, which receive fluid, called lymph, from the extracellular compartment.
—lymph passes through increasingly larger lymphatic vessels and through the lymphoid organs, which filter it and add lymphocytes and other constituents before returning it to the blood vascular system.

Blood Vascular System

Heart
—a four-chambered muscular organ composed of two atria and two ventricles.
—is surrounded by a fibrous sac, the pericardium, whose innermost layer is known as the epicardium.
—possesses an internal fibrous skeleton and a three-layered wall, composed of epicardium, myocardium, and endocardium.

Pericardium
—is the sac-like structure enclosing the heart. The outer layer of this sac, the parietal pericardium, is composed of fibrous connective tissue; the inner layer, the visceral pericardium (also known as epicardium), is reflected on the wall of the heart.

Epicardium
—the outermost layer covering the heart (the visceral pericardium).
—is composed of a simple squamous epithelium (mesothelium) overlying a thin layer

of fibroelastic connective tissue. Deep to this is an adipose tissue containing the coronary vessels and nerves.

Myocardium

—the thick muscular wall of the heart.

—consists of layers of cardiac muscle cells arranged in a spiral fashion about the heart chambers and inserted into the fibrous skeleton.

—its contractions propel blood into the arteries for distribution to the body tissues.

Cardiac Muscle Cells

—perform contractile functions.

—modified cardiac muscle cells are responsible for generating and conducting the electrical impulses that regulate the heartbeat. (See Chapter 6 for a description of histologic features of cardiac muscle cells.)

Fibrous Skeleton of Heart

—consists of thick collagen fibers arranged in various directions.

—fibrocartilage is also located in various regions of the fibrous skeleton.

Endocardium

—the layer lining the lumen of the heart.

—is continuous with the intima of the vessels leaving and entering the heart.

—is composed of simple squamous epithelium (endothelium) lying on a thin layer of loose connective tissue containing elastic and collagen fibers and occasional smooth muscle cells.

—subendocardial layer (lying deep to endocardium) is connective tissue where veins, nerves, and Purkinje fibers are located.

Cardiac Valves

—are interposed between the atrial and the ventricular chambers.

Atrioventricular Valves

—are composed of a skeleton of fibrous connective tissue, arranged like an aponeurosis and attached to the anuli fibrosi of the cardiac skeleton.

—are covered by endothelium and possess a core of subendothelially derived connective tissue.

Impulse-Generating System

—is composed of several specialized structures, including the sinoatrial node, atrioventricular node, and atrioventricular bundle of His.

—its coordinated interactions regulate the heartbeat.

Sinoatrial Node

—"pacemaker" of the heart, is composed of specialized cardiac muscle cells (smaller than the typical cardiac muscle cells) that initiate contraction of the heart.

—its cells, located in the sinoatrial node of the right atrial wall, contain few myofibrils and are arranged in concentric rings.

—impulses generated at the sinoatrial node activate cardiac muscle cells in the atrial walls, and the impulse is conducted to the atrioventricular node.

Atrioventricular Node

—is located in the wall of the interventricular septum between the septal leaf of the tricuspid valve and the opening of the coronary sinus.

—is similar to the sinoatrial node, in that it is composed of a meshwork of modified, smaller than normal cardiac muscle cells (containing fewer myofibrils) interwoven with connective tissue.

—also contains adipose tissue and is richly supplied by large arterioles.

Atrioventricular Bundle of His

—a band of conducting tissue radiating out from the atrioventricular node to the muscle cells in the ventricles.

—is composed of specialized, large, modified cardiac muscle cells, Purkinje fibers, that branch into right and left bundles.

—left bundle subdivides as it reaches the apex of the heart and sends out collaterals, which make contact with the contractile cardiac muscle cells via gap junctions. (See Chapter 6 for histologic descriptions of the cells of the Purkinje fibers.)

Autonomic Nerves

—modulate the rhythm of the heartbeat.

—parasympathetic nerves, carried by the vagus nerve to the sinoatrial node, slow the heartbeat.

—sympathetic nerves, derived from several sources, accelerate the heartbeat.

Arteries

—conduct blood away from the heart.

—possess walls composed of three layers: tunica intima, tunica media, and tunica adventitia.

  —tunica intima: (innermost layer) lines the lumen of the vessel.
  —tunica media: (middle layer) is composed primarily of several layers of smooth muscle cells.
  —tunica adventitia: (outermost layer) consists of fibroelastic connective tissue that, in larger vessels, contains vasa vasorum (vessels of the vessel).

—elastic (conducting) arteries are the largest arteries and leave the heart proper.

—muscular (distributing) arteries deliver blood to the organs.

—arterioles, smallest of the arteries, regulate blood flow into the capillary beds.

Elastic Arteries

—include the aorta and its large branches.

—are composed of three layers: the tunicae intima, media, and adventitia.

Tunica Intima

—composed of a layer of endothelial cells (a simple squamous epithelium) overlying a subendothelial layer composed of loose connective tissue containing fibroblasts, collagen, and elastic fibers.

—elastic fibers form an incomplete internal elastic lamina, interlaced with smooth muscle cells.

Endothelial Cells

—are polygonal with pinocytotic vesicles, rough endoplasmic reticulum, microfilaments, lysosomes, and intercellular junctions.

—house rod-like inclusions (Weibel-Palade bodies) that may store factor VIII, a coagulating component synthesized by these cells.

Figure 8.1. Photomicrograph of a muscular artery (*below*) and its companion vein (*above*). × 132. (From Gartner LP, Hiatt JL: *Atlas of Histology*. Baltimore, Williams & Wilkins, 1987.)

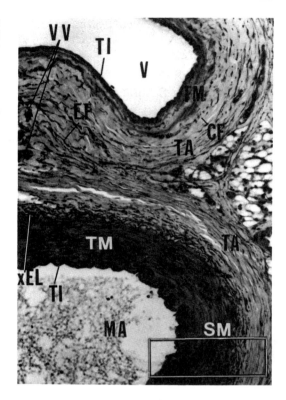

Tunica Media

—(middle layer of an elastic artery) is composed of elastic fibers layered in 40 to 70 fenestrated membranes (whose layers increase with age).

—also contain (interspersed between the elastic laminae) smooth muscle cells, collagen fibers, and ground substance (mostly chondroitin sulfate).

—external elastic laminae are thin and inconspicuous.

Tunica Adventitia

—the thin outer layer of an elastic artery, consisting of fibroblasts, collagen, and elastic fibers that form a loose network, as well as vasa vasorum.

—vasa vasorum, small vessels that supply the artery, are present and may penetrate the tunica media for some distance.

—lymphatic vessels are also located in the adventitia.

Muscular Arteries

—the distributing arteries, which are the most abundant type in the body.

Tunica Intima

—thinner than that in most elastic arteries; consists of an endothelium, subendothelial connective tissue, and an internal elastic lamina.

—endothelium conforms to the contour of the internal elastic lamina (which is often contracted in fixed tissue).

—subendothelial connective tissue layer lacks smooth muscle cells.

—internal elastic lamina is well developed, appears refractile with hematoxylin and eosin stain, but is clearly defined by an elastic stain. Occasionally it is doubled.

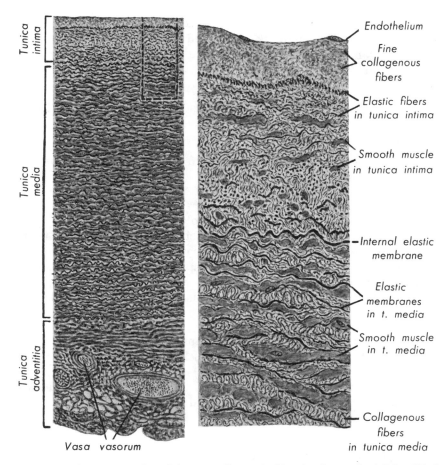

Figure 8.2. Diagram of a cross section of the ascending aorta. The drawing on the *left* (× 60) displays the entire thickness of the vessel. *Boxed area* is shown at a higher magnification (× 285). (From Copenhaver WM, Bunge RP, Bunge MB: *Bailey's Textbook of Histology*, ed 16. Baltimore, Williams & Wilkins, 1971.)

Tunica Media
—is composed of many (up to 40) layers of smooth muscle cells arranged in a circular or helical fashion and interspersed with elastic fibers.
—number of muscle cell layers is related to the size of the artery, and a thick external elastic lamina defines the outermost layer of the media.

Tunica Adventitia
—contains a variety of connective tissue cells as well as collagenous and elastic fibers.
—also contains vasa vasorum and lymphatic vessels.

Arterioles
—smallest arteries have a diameter of less than 0.1 mm. The thickness of the vessel wall approximates the diameter of the lumen.

Tunica Intima
—is composed of a continuous layer of endothelial cells whose nuclei bulge into the lumen.

—endothelial cells contain Weibel-Palade bodies.

—subendothelial connective tissue is sparse and contains a few reticular fibers.

—internal elastic lamina is absent, but in some of the larger arterioles a few elastic fibers are present.

Tunica Media

—consists of one or two layers of smooth muscle cells wrapped helically around the intima.

Tunica Adventitia

—is composed of loose connective tissue with a few fibers, connective tissue cells, and unmyelinated nerves.

Metarterioles

—the branched vessels that derive from arterioles.

—possess a discontinuous layer of smooth muscle cells (tunica media) that can exert some control over blood flow into the capillary network beyond them.

—a complete ring of muscle, the precapillary sphincter encircles the capillary about its origin from the metarteriole.

—precapillary sphincter contractions control blood flow into the capillary bed.

Innervation

—arteries are innervated by unmyelinated sympathetic fibers that are responsible for vasoconstriction, but arteries of skeletal muscle also contain cholinergic (parasympathetic) fibers that initiate vasodilation.

—special sensory nerve endings in the walls of the arteries include the carotid sinus (which acts as a baroreceptor for stretch) and the carotid and aortic bodies (which serve as chemoreceptors).

Carotid Sinus

—a dilatation located at the bifurcation of the common carotid artery, consisting of a thickened area of the adventitia that possesses sensory nerve endings derived from the glossopharyngeal nerve.

—its thin media responds easily to stretch, which stimulates the receptor and initiates a nerve reflex that modifies systemic blood pressure.

—a few baroreceptors are found elsewhere in the body but are less easily identified.

Carotid Bodies

—are located in the wall of the common carotid artery as it bifurcates into the external and internal carotid arteries.

—are flat, richly innervated structures served by the glossopharyngeal and vagus nerves.

—contain groups of epithelioid cells of two types, type I and type II cells.

Type I (Glomus) Cells

—possess dense-cored vesicles and occur in clusters that are surrounded by type II (sheath) cells.

—are of two subtypes, type A and type B.

—type A cells are more numerous, possess few processes, and have twice as many dense-cored vesicles as type B cells.

—type B cells are characterized by long thin processes. These cells may function as chemoreceptors, modulators, or as paracrine cells.

Type II (Sheath) Cells
—surround the type I glomus cells.
—aortic bodies located in the aorta and subclavian arteries are chemoreceptor organs.

Histophysiology

Elastic Arteries
—which receive blood directly from the heart, tend to absorb the pressure created by each heartbeat, due to the expansion of the thick elastic laminae.
—rebound to maintain pressure as the pressure ebbs during diastole.

Muscular Arteries
—are responsible for delivering blood to body organs. The volumes delivered are determined by neural control and local conditions, but aging alters the intima and media and affects vascular function.

Aneurysm
—occurs due to a weakness in the wall of an artery. A ballooning out occurs and the vessel may burst.

Atherosclerosis
—a disease of arteries brought about through a series of events, beginning with injury to the endothelium and accumulation of monocytes (from blood) and smooth muscle cells (from the media) in the subendothelial connective tissue of the intima.
—factors are released by the endothelium, macrophages, and smooth muscle cells (as well as platelets) that stimulate the smooth muscle cells to divide and produce extracellular products.
—extracellular products accumulate, along with lipid, in the intima so that an atherosclerotic plaque is formed.
—plaque may completely occlude the lumen of the vessel, blocking blood flow and resulting in a heart attack.

Capillaries

—the small vessels located between terminal arterioles and the venules.
—average diameter is 8 to 10 μm; length ranges from 0.25 to 1 mm (except those located in the adrenal cortex and renal medulla, which are considerably longer).
—are basically endothelial tubes composed of one layer of endothelial cells, resting on a basal lamina and formed into a hollow cylinder, and associated pericytes.

Pericytes
—mesenchymal-like multipotential cells with long processes that are associated with capillaries at certain sites.
—usually share the basal lamina of the endothelium.

Endothelial Cells
—polygonal and oriented with their long axes in the direction of blood flow.
—size ranges from 10 to 30 μm, and because their cytoplasm is attenuated, their nucleus bulges into the lumen.
—at the margins the cells may be only 0.2 μm thick.
—their organelles (as revealed by electron micrographs) include Golgi apparatus near the nucleus, free ribosomes, mitochondria, and some rough endoplasmic reticulum.

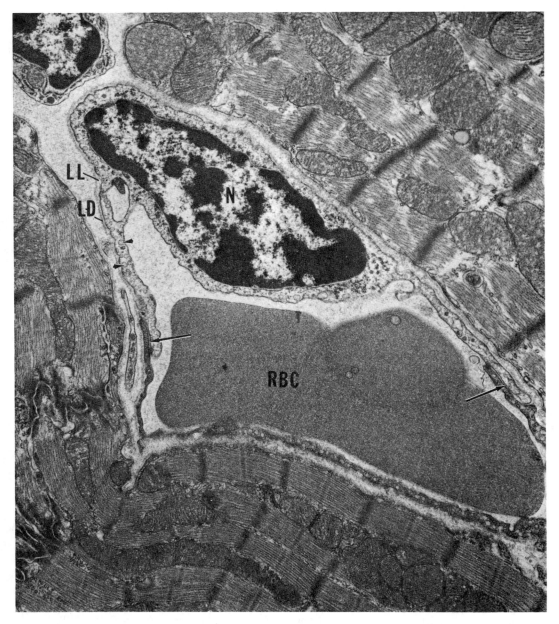

Figure 8.3. Electron micrograph of a continuous capillary in heart muscle. The nucleus **(N)** of the endothelial cell bulges into the lumen occupied by an erythrocyte (red blood cell, **RBC**). **LD**, lamina densa; **LL**, lamina (lucida). × 29,330. (From Gartner LP, Hiatt JL: *Atlas of Histology*. Baltimore, Williams & Wilkins, 1987.)

—filaments, (9 to 11 nm diameter) observed in the perinuclear zone may represent vimentin and be supportive in function.
—fascia occludents normally present: its complexity is related to physiological permeability of the particular capillary.

Capillary Types

Continuous (Somatic) Capillaries

—possess an endothelium that forms a continuous uninterrupted layer around the entire capillary.

—are located in nervous tissue, muscle, connective tissue, and exocrine glands.

—occluding junctions in continuous capillaries are responsible for providing the blood-brain barrier, although they may permit the passage of small molecules.

—pinocytotic vesicles (up to 70 nm diameter) permit transport in both directions (although they are absent in nervous tissue).

Fenestrated (Visceral) Capillaries

—possess an endothelium that lies on a basal lamina and displays large fenestrae (60 to 80 nm diameter) spanned by a diaphragm.

—their morphology is related to their abilities to exchange fluid and macromolecules rapidly.

Diaphragms

—closing these fenestrae do not possess the typical unit membrane structure but are filamentous.

—are absent in some fenestrated capillaries, such as those of the renal glomerulus, which possess thick basal laminae.

Discontinuous (Sinusoidal) Capillaries

—are characterized by an endothelium (containing multiple fenestrae without diaphragms) and a discontinuous basal lamina.

—have a large diameter (up to 40 μm) and exhibit a tortuous course.

—are located in the liver and hemopoietic organs.

Function

—capillaries function in selective permeability, permitting the exchange of oxygen, carbon dioxide, metabolites, and other substances between the blood and the tissues.

Permeability

—is regulated by the morphology of the endothelium lining the capillary and by the size, shape, and charge of the individual molecule.

—some substances diffuse or are actively transported across the cell membrane, while others pass through the intercellular junctions and/or fenestrae.

—leukocytes leave the bloodstream by squeezing through the junctions between endothelial cells, a process called diapedesis.

Histamine and Bradykinin

—alter capillary permeability when they are released locally, and in this way the capillary plays a role promoting the inflammatory response.

—capillary endothelial cells have the capacity to metabolize certain substrates.

—convert angiotensin I to angiotensin II in the lung.

—deactivate bradykinin, serotonin, prostaglandins, norepinephrine, and thrombin, etc., as well as break down triglycerides and cholesterol.

—release prostacyclin (prostaglandin I_2), which inhibits platelet aggregation and clot formation.

Blood Flow

—into the capillary bed is controlled by two different mechanisms.

Terminal Arterioles
—have a luminal diameter of 30 to 50 μm and only a single layer of smooth muscle in their media.
—deliver blood either to true capillaries or to metarterioles (having precapillary sphincters).

True Capillaries
—may arise from the proximal portion of the metarteriole, and blood flow into them tois controlled by precapillary sphincters.
—also drain into the portion distal to the metarteriole (thoroughfare channels).

Thoroughfare Channels
—serve as a bypass for blood flow when capillary beds are closed by the precapillary sphincters. This occurs in regions such as the skin and the ear, where thermoregulation is important.
—deliver their blood to small venules.

Veins

—return blood to the heart.
—begin as venules (small vessels at the terminal ends of the capillaries), which increase in size and become continuous with small veins, medium-sized veins, and finally large veins.

Venules
—small vessels with a diameter of 0.2 to 1 mm, whose walls are composed of three layers: the tunicae intima, media, and adventitia.
—possess biological functions similar to capillaries.
—tunica intima is composed of endothelial cells.
—tunica media contains one or two layers of smooth muscle cells.
—tunica adventitia (the thickest layer), is composed of several layers of collagen fibers.

Small and Medium Veins
—the most common in the body.
—diameters range from 1 to 9 mm; they possess three layers in their walls: tunicae intima, media, and adventitia.
—tunica intima contains endothelial cells and occasionally a thin subendothelial connective tissue layer.
—tunica media contains small bundles of smooth muscle interspersed with reticular fibers and a network of elastic fibers.
—tunica adventitia is composed of many layers of collagen fibers interspersed with fibroblasts.

Veins
—may possess valves in their lumina that act to prevent retrograde flow of the blood.
—valves are composed of a core of elastic connective tissue lined by endothelium.

Large Veins
—include the major collecting blood vessels of the abdominal cavity and those leading directly into the heart.

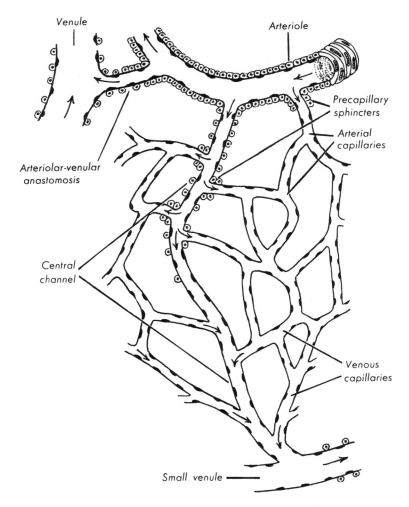

Figure 8.4. Schematic diagram of a capillary bed, demonstrating the central channel with its two subdivisions, the muscular metarteriole and the thoroughfare channel. (From Kelly DE, Wood RL, Enders AC: *Bailey's Textbook of Microscopic Anatomy*, ed 18. Baltimore, Williams & Wilkins, 1984.)

—possess a well-developed intima, a thin media with smooth muscle cells, and a thick well-developed adventitia.
—of the abdominal cavity contain bundles of longitudinally oriented smooth muscle cells in the adventitia that apparently assist in preventing distension of the vessel.
—entering the heart, possess cardiac muscle fibers in their adventitia as they approach the heart.

Lymphatic Vascular System

—consists of vessels in the connective tissue that collect excess tissue fluid, called lymph, and return it to the venous system.

Lymphatic Vessels

—drain most tissues, with the exception of the nervous system and the bone marrow.

Lymphatic Capillaries

—thin-walled vessels that begin as blind-ended channels.
—are composed of a single layer of attenuated endothelial cells (lacking both fenestrations and zonula occludentes) but held patent by fine anchoring filaments that extend into the connective tissue.
—their basal lamina is very sparse.

Large Lymphatic Vessels

—are similar to venules in structure except that they have larger lumina.
—their thin walls make it difficult to distinguish the various tunics, but lymph flow is controlled by valves in their lumina.
—converge and interposed along their routes are lymph nodes that filter the lymph before it is returned to the blood. (See Chapter 9 for a description of histologic features of the lymph nodes.)

Lymphatic Ducts

—possess a morphology similar to that of veins.
—contain a longitudinal and circular layer of smooth muscle cells in their media.
—their adventitia is poorly developed and contains vasa vasorum and nerves.

REVIEW TESTS
CIRCULATORY SYSTEM

DIRECTIONS: *One* or *more* of the given completions or answers is/are correct. Choose answer:

A. if only **1,2,** and **3** are correct
B. if only **1** and **3** are correct
C. if only **2** and **4** are correct
D. of only **4** is correct
E. if **all** are correct

8.1. The pericardium
1. is a sac-like structure enclosing the heart
2. has a fibrous layer and a serous layer
3. is reflected on the heart as the epicardium
4. accumulates fat in its visceral layer

8.2. The myocardium
1. is the muscular wall of the heart
2. contains two types of muscle cells
3. contains cardiac muscle tissue inserted into a fibrous skeleton
4. lines the lumen of the heart

8.3. The impulse-generating system of the heart includes the following:
1. atrioventricular node
2. sinoatrial node
3. atrioventricular bundle of His
4. sympathetic nerves

8.4. The tunica media of elastic arteries and muscular arteries differ primarily in that
1. elastic arteries contain only elastic fibers
2. the external elastic lamina of muscular arteries is prominent
3. muscular arteries contain only muscle fibers
4. the relative amounts of elastic fibers and muscle fibers differ in each type of artery

8.5. Metarterioles
1. drain into venules
2. possess an incomplete smooth muscle cell layer around the vessel
3. receive blood from thoroughfare channels
4. precede the precapillary sphincter

DIRECTIONS: Each of the following questions contains four suggested answers. Choose the *one best* response to each question.

8.6. The carotid sinus
a. lies in the bifurcation of the common carotid artery and acts as a chemoreceptor
b. measures oxygen concentration in the blood
c. initiates a nerve reflex that modifies blood pressure
d. is a modification of the tunica intima within the bifurcation of the common carotid artery

8.7. Capillary types are based on
a. the presence of fenestrae
b. fasciae occludentes
c. the absence of fenestrae
d. all of the above

8.8. Capillaries found in the central nervous system are without pinocytotic vesicles and are examples of
a. continuous (somatic) capillaries
b. fenestrated (visceral) capillaries
c. sinusoidal capillaries
d. none of the above

8.9. Capillaries function in all of the following *except*
a. exchange of metabolites
b. exchange of gases
c. control of blood pressure
d. inhibiting clot formation

8.10. Large veins of the abdominal cavity possess
a. no true endothelial layer
b. a longitudinal smooth muscle layer
c. a poorly developed tunica intima layer
d. no tunica adventitia

DIRECTIONS: The following terms refer to the photomicrograph (Fig. 8.5). The letters on the figure correspond to the numbered items appearing below the photomicrograph. For each numbered item, select the *one* letter that *best* corresponds to that item. Each letter may be used once, more than once, or not at all.

Figure 8.5. From Gartner LP, Hiatt JL: *Atlas of Histology*. Baltimore, Williams & Wilkins, 1987.)

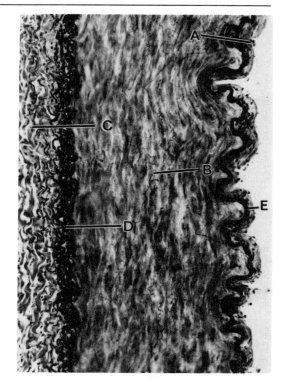

8.11. Tunica media

8.12. External elastic lamina

8.13. Endothelium

8.14. Tunica adventitia

8.15. Internal elastic lamina

ANSWERS AND EXPLANATIONS
CIRCULATORY SYSTEM

8.1. E (all answers are correct)
The pericardium is a sac-like structure consisting of an outer fibrous layer and an inner serous layer. It is reflected upon the heart to become the epicardium, where fat is accumulated.

8.2. B (1 and 3)
The myocardium is the muscular layer of the heart that contains cardiac muscle cells. The muscle tissue is inserted into the fibrous skeleton of the heart. It does not line the lumen nor does it comprise the cardiac valves.

8.3. A (1, 2, and 3)
The impulse-generating system of the heart includes the sinoatrial node, atrioventricular node, and the atrioventricular bundle of His. While the sympathetic nerves act to modulate the system, they neither initiate nor generate the impulse to the heart.

8.4. C (2 and 4)
The tunica media of elastic arteries and muscular arteries both contain elastic fibers and muscle fibers. However, as their name implies, elastic arteries contain more elastic fibers than muscular arteries, and vice versa. The external elastic lamina of muscular arteries is also prominent.

8.5. C (2 and 4)
Metarterioles are the branched terminal ends of the arteriole system. They are characterized by a single incomplete layer of smooth muscle cells. The precapillary sphincter lies distal to the metarteriole. Thoroughfare channels drain the metarteriole.

8.6. C
The carotid sinus lies in the bifurcation of the common carotid artery and acts as a baroreceptor. Its adventitia is enlarged and receives fibers from the glossopharyngeal nerve. When stretched the nerve endings initiate a reflex that modifies blood pressure.

8.7. D
Capillary types are based on the structure of their endothelial cells and the presence or absence of a basal lamina.

8.8. A
Capillaries located in the central nervous system are without fenestrae and pinocytotic vesicles and have true occluding junctions, thus accounting for the blood-brain barrier. Thus only continuous capillaries are located in the central nervous tissues.

8.9. C
Capillaries function as the exchange vessels for metabolites and gases and in inhibiting clot formation. Capillaries do not control blood pressure.

8.10. B
Large veins of the abdominal cavity contain longitudinal muscles in their tunica adventitia, which prevents distension of the vessel. The vein morphology is much like that of an artery, therefore it contains all the tunics.

8.11. Tunica media (**B**)

8.12. External elastic lamina (**D**)

8.13. Endothelium (**A**)

8.14. Tunica adventitia (**C**)

8.15. Internal elastic lamina (**E**)

9
Lymphatic Tissue

Organization of Lymphatic Tissue

—lymphatic tissue is organized into nodular and diffuse accumulations that act in concert to defend the body against foreign elements.
—the basis of this defense is the immune system, which depends on the actions of two principal cell types, the lymphocytes and macrophages.

Lymphocytes

—include the T and B lymphocytes, also referred to as T and B cells (and their various subtypes), as well as the natural killer (NK) and killer (K) cells.
—clones of T and B cells are established around the time of birth. Clones are small numbers of identical cells; each clone has the ability to recognize and combat a single (or a small group of closely related) antigen.
—T lymphocytes acquire both immunological competency and surface markers (which assist them in their functions) in the thymus; they are responsible for the cellularly mediated responses, e.g., graft rejection phenomena.
—B lymphocytes most probably acquire immunological competency and surface markers in the bone marrow; these cells are responsible for the humorally mediated responses.
—potentiation of B lymphocytes in birds occurs in the bursa of Fabricius, a diverticulum of the cloaca (not present in mammals).

Cells of the Immune System

Lymphocytes

T Lymphocytes

—are responsible for cellularly mediated immune response. They possess Fc fragment as well as immunoglobulin-like receptors on the external aspect of their plasma membranes.

Immunoglobulin-Like Receptors

—have not been characterized; each one is believed to have specificity to only one antigen. There are several subtypes of T lymphocytes.

T-Helper (Inducer) Cells

—subtypes of T lymphocytes that assist B cells in initiating a humoral response.
—initiation occurs either by establishing physical contact with the B cell or more

frequently by producing releasing factors, known as lymphokines, that trigger B cells to respond to the antigenic stimulus.

Thymic-Dependent Antigens
—require T cell intermediaries that facilitate the occurrence of a response.

Thymic-Independent Antigens
—may be combated by B cells without the intermediary action of T-helper cells.

T-helper Cells
—also activate macrophages, T-memory cells, T-cytotoxic cells, T-suppressor cells, and perhaps even fibroblasts, CFU-Ly, and CFU-S cells.
—bear IgM receptors on their external cell surface.

T-Suppressor Cells
—function in modulating the extent of the humoral response by controlling the actions of the T-helper cells.
—bear IgG receptors on their plasma membranes and control the activities of other types of T cells.

T-Memory cells
—are long-lived, committed, immunocompetent stem cells that are formed during proliferation in response to an antigenic challenge.
—they do not react against the antigen but remain in circulation (or in specific regions of the lymphatic tissue).
—they thus increase the size of the original clone and thereby provide a faster, secondary response against a future challenge by the same antigen.

T-Cytotoxic Cells
—are also known as T-killer cells. Once they have become sensitized (probably by T-helper cells), they lyse foreign cells whose antigens they recognize.

Lymphokines
—are regulatory proteins manufactured and released by T lymphocytes, which modulate the activities of the various cells participating in the immune response.
—include chemotactic agents for granulocytes and macrophages.
—include agents that inhibit migration of neutrophils (NIF) and macrophages (MIF).
—include substances that activate (or suppress) the activities of certain cells, e.g., macrophage-activating factor (MAF) and interferon (an activator of NK cells).
—include agents that permit long-term growth of T lymphocytes (interleukin 2), neutrophils, and macrophages (colony-stimulating factor, CSF).
—include substances that may activate fibroblasts to manufacture collagen. This is only a partial list of the many functions of lymphokines.

B Lymphocytes
—synthesize a small quantity of immunoglobulins that remain attached to the external aspect of their plasma membrane.
—are fully immunocompetent and have the capability of responding to an antigenic stimulus. They participate in the humoral immune response.
—are specific against particular antigenic determinants.

Antigenic Challenge

—causes B cells (usually prompted by T-helper cells) to undergo mitotic activity, to produce B cells bearing the same antigenic determinants.

—majority of new B cells become transformed into plasma cells, which function in antibody synthesis (discussed in Chapter 3), but the remainder will become B-memory cells.

B-Memory Cells

—arise during an antigenic challenge but do not become transformed into plasma cells.

—remain either in circulation or occupy preferential positions in lymphatic tissues, thus increasing the size of their clone and enhancing the severity and rapidity of a secondary response.

NK (Natural Killer) Cells

—belong to the null cell population, since they bear no surface determinants.

—are similar to T lymphocytes, in that they are cytotoxic, but differ from T cells in that they are not potentiated by and can develop in the absence of the thymus.

K Cells (Killer Cells)

—an additional population of lymphocytes (also members of the null cell population) that bear no surface determinants.

—may be a subtype of (or the same as) NK cells, since neither requires potentiation by the thymus.

—possess Fc receptors on the external aspect of their plasma membranes and recognize and bind to IgG on foreign cells.

—bound K cells lyse the foreign cell, a reaction known as antibody-dependent cellular cytotoxicity (ADCC).

Macrophages

Structure and functions of macrophages were discussed in Chapter 3, but their activities in the immune response were not detailed there. Some authors contend that another group of cells, lymphoid dendritic cells (e.g., Langerhans cells, follicular dendritic cells, M cells), rather than macrophages, interact with immunocompetent cells and antigens to elicit an immune response. In this review book, antigen-presenting cells and macrophages are considered to belong to the same population of cells.

Functions of Macrophages

—phagocytose, degrade, and process antigens and present the modified antigens (known as immunogens) to T lymphocytes. These immunogens have an increased effectiveness in initiating the immune response.

—release interleukin 1, a substance that stimulates mitotic activity of T lymphocytes, as well as colony-stimulating factors (CSF), a substance that promotes granulopoiesis.

—secrete prostaglandins (PGE_2), which have the ability to decrease certain immune responses.

Interferon and MAF

—produced by T-lymphocytes, activate macrophages so that they become avidly phagocytic and cytotoxic.

—cytotoxic abilities of macrophages are related to the antibody coating of the target cell, a process referred to as an ADCC reaction.

Immunoglobulins

—antibodies that are specific against one or a few closely related antigens.
—are composed of two heavy and two light polypeptide chains that are held together by disulfide linkages. It has been estimated that human serum contains over 100 million different immunoglobulin molecules.
—have regions that are identical to those of all other immunoglobulin molecules (constant region), as well as regions that are different from those of all other molecules (variable region).
—variable regions determine the specificity of the molecule against the antigenic determinant of a particular antigen.
—extremely large antigens, such as a microorganism, have numerous antigenic determinants, thus evoking a complex immune response.

Human Serum

—contains five principal types of heavy chains, determining five different classes of immunoglobulins, each of which is designated by a letter of the alphabet.

Immunoglobulin A (IgA)

—is found both in the bloodstream and in glandular secretions.
—within the vascular system IgA exists in its monomeric form (two heavy and two light chains).
—in glandular secretions IgA forms a dimer coupled to a secretory component protein.
—functions to combat antigens on the surface of the body.

Immunoglobulin D (IgD)

—is a monomer attached to the external aspect of the lymphocyte plasmalemma. Although its function is not known it is believed to be an antigen receptor.

Immunoglobulin (IgE)

—is a monomer that preferentially binds to the external aspect of the plasmalemmae of mast cells and basophils.
—during an antigenic challenge, the antigens become attached to the IgE, which causes the mast cells and basophils to degranulate.
—this degranulation releases the pharmacologic agents heparin, histamine, eosinophil chemotactic factor of anaphylaxis (ECF-A), and the slow-reacting substance of anaphylaxis (SRS-A).

Immunoglobulin G (IgG)

—the most common type of immunoglobulin, is a monomer (composed of two heavy and two light chains).
—constitutes most of the immunoglobulins found in the bloodstream.
—binds to invading microorganisms and various toxins.
—functions in complement fixation and becomes attached to the Fc receptors of macrophages. IgG is able to cross the placental barrier.

Immunoglobulin M (IgM)

—the first antibody formed in an antigenic challenge. It is a pentamer (having five pairs of heavy and light chains attached to each other) whose large size imparts it with potent antibacterial characteristics.

Diffuse Lymphatic Tissue

—is especially prominent in the loose connective tissue deep to wet epithelia, such as in the lamina propria of the intestine, where immunological protection is required for bacterial, antigenic, and/or toxic challenges.

—organized as scattered clusters of lymphoid cells or as lymphatic nodules.

Lymphatic Nodules

—transitory, dense spherical accumulations of lymphocytes (mostly B cells).

—present frequently a central lightly stained area, the germinal center, composed of medium and large lymphocytes (lymphoblasts), indicative of active cell division and transformation of B cells into plasma cells.

Corona

—the peripheral, dark region is composed mostly of small, newly formed lymphocytes.

Aggregates

—of lymphatic nodules, known as Peyers's patches, are found in the ileum and are discussed in Chapter 14.

Lymph Nodes

—are small, encapsulated, ovoid- to kidney-shaped organs that are scattered along lymphatic vessels throughout the body, although they are more concentrated in the neck, axilla, and groin.

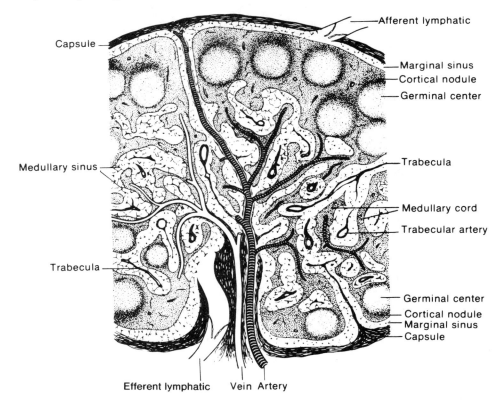

9.1. Diagram of a lymph node. (From Kelly DE, Wood RL, Enders AC: *Bailey's Textbook of Microscopic Anatomy*, ed. 18. Baltimore, Williams & Wilkins, 1984.)

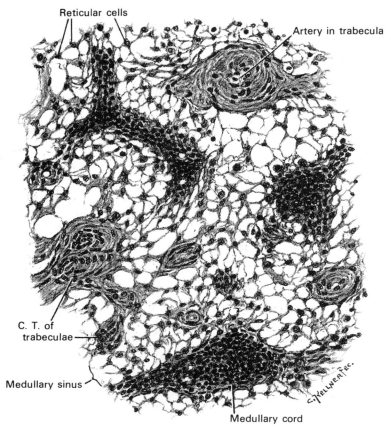

Reticular cells

Artery in trabecula

C. T. of
trabeculae

Medullary sinus

Medullary cord

Figure 9.2. Diagram of a section of the medulla of a lymph node. *C.T.*, connective tissue. (From Copenhaver WM, Bunge RP, Bunge MB: *Bailey's Textbook of Histology*, ed 16. Baltimore, Williams & Wilkins, 1971.)

—filter the lymph and produce lymphocytes.

General Structure

—a connective tissue capsule surrounds the entire node, which is divided into a cortex and a medulla.

—convex surface of the lymph node receives afferent lymphatic vessels.

—concave aspect (hilus) is where efferent lymphatic vessels and venules leave and arterioles enter the lymph mode.

Capsule

—usually surrounded by adipose tissue, is composed of dense irregular collagenous connective tissue that sends septae into the substance of the node.

—afferent lymphatic vessels that pierce the convex aspect of the capsule possess valves that impose a unidirectional flow of lymph throughout the node.

Cortex

—is deep to the capsule but is absent at the hilus. It is incompletely subdivided into smaller, intercommunicating compartments by connective tissue septa derived from the capsule.

—contains three major constituents, lymphatic nodules, sinusoids, and the paracortex.

Lymphatic Nodules

—(some with germinal centers) are composed mainly of B lymphocytes, few T lymphocytes, antigen-presenting cells (follicular dendritic cells), macrophages, and reticular cells.

Sinusoids

—are endothelially lined spaces that extend along the capsule and trabeculae and are known as subcapsular and cortical (paratrabecular) sinuses, respectively.

Paracortex

—is composed of non-nodular arrangement of T lymphocytes (the thymus-dependent area of the lymph node).
—circulating lymphocytes gain access to lymph nodes via postcapillary venules (recognized by their cuboidal-shaped endothelia) in the paracortex.

Medulla

—is surrounded by the cortex except at the region of the hilus.
—is composed of medullary sinusoids and medullary cords.

Medullary Sinusoids

—are endothelially lined spaces housing reticular cells (whose processes frequently span the sinusoids, retarding and causing turbulence in the lymph flow) and macrophages (or their processes).
—receive lymph from the cortical sinuses.

Medullary Cords

—are composed of lymphocytes and plasma cells, many of which migrated from the cortex to enter sinusoids of the medulla.

Reticular Fibers

—compose a network of fibers that constitute the framework of the lymph node.
—network of fibers is intimately associated with the capsule and the trabeculae of the lymph node. The reticulum is more tightly woven in the cortex than in the medulla.

Function of Lymph Nodes

—is to filter lymph and maintain and produce T and B lymphocytes. Moreover, memory cells (especially T cells) are preferentially located in lymph nodes.

Thymus

—unlike most lymphatic organs, is dervied both from endoderm (third pharyngeal pouch gives rise to its epithelial primordium) and mesoderm (lymphocytes).
—is located in the superior mediastinum, just superior to the pericardium.
—begins to involute near the time of puberty.
—is composed of two lobes, subdivided into incomplete lobules, that are separated into cortex and medulla, neither of which contains lymphatic nodules.
—lobules are enveloped by connective tissue septa that arise from the connective tissue capsule of the organ.

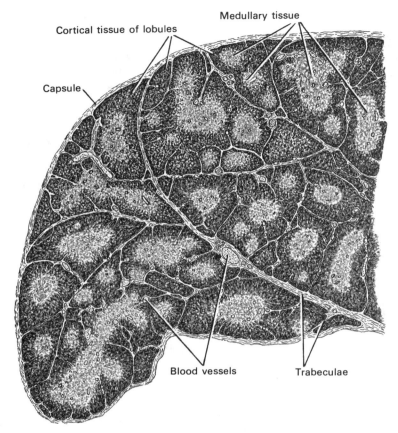

Cortical tissue of lobules

Medullary tissue

Capsule

Blood vessels

Trabeculae

9.3. Diagram of a section of the thymus at birth. (From Kelly DE, Wood RL, Enders AC: *Bailey's Textbook of Microscopic Anatomy*, ed 18. Baltimore, Williams & Wilkins, 1984.)

Cortex

Septa

—are composed of delicate collagen fibers derived from the slender capsule of the thymus.

—form an incomplete investment around the periphery of each lobule.

—small arterioles within the septa originate from vessels in the capsule and provide capillary loops that enter the substance of the cortex.

Epithelial Reticular Cells

—are derived from the third pharyngeal pouch.

—are pale cells, with a large, ovoid, lightly staining nucleus that often displays a nucleolus.

—possess long processes that completely surround the cortex, isolating it both from the connective tissue septa and from the medulla of the thymus.

—processes, filled with bundles of tonofilaments, form desmosomal contacts with each other.

Granules

—within cytoplasm of epithelial reticular cells are believed to contain secretory products, such as thymosin, serum thymic factor, and thymopoietin.
—these substances function in the potentiation of CFU-LyT, transforming them into immunocompetent T cells.

T Lymphocytes (Thymocytes)

—occur in large numbers within the cortex.
—are in the process of differentiation.

Medium and Large Lymphocytes (Lymphoblasts)

—are present deep to the epithelial reticular cells at the periphery of the cortex. During maturation, T cells are surrounded by processes of epithelial reticular cells, segregating them from antigens.

Maturing T Cells

—migrate toward the medulla to be released; however, most of the T cells produced die in the cortex and are phagocytosed by macrophages.

Vascularization

—is composed solely of continuous capillaries that are completely surrounded by reticular epithelial cells.
—the intervening space is occupied by the basal laminae of the endothelial and epithelial reticular cells and by macrophages, establishing the blood-thymus barrier.
—macrophages ensure that antigens escaping from the vascular supply do not reach the developing T cells in the cortex.

Medulla

Cells

—are mainly fully mature T cells and numerous epithelial reticular cells, many of which form whorl-like accretions, known as Hassall's (thymic) corpuscles (of unknown function), some of whose cells display various stages of keratinization (or even calcification).
—incidence of Hassall's corpuscles increases as a function of age.

Lymphocytes

—are loosely packed in the medulla, which, therefore, appears lighter stained than does the cortex. Also the medulla of one lobule is continuous with that of the other lobules.

Vascularization

—is supplied by arterioles and venules. The medulla does not possess a blood-thymus barrier, and it is here that T lymphocytes enter venules (and efferent lymphatic vessels) to exit the thymus.

Function

—to stimulate proliferation and potentiation of CFU-LyT cells (present in the cortex) so they become immunocompetent T lymphocytes, which enter venules or efferent lymph vessels of the medulla and become distributed to the thymic-dependent re-

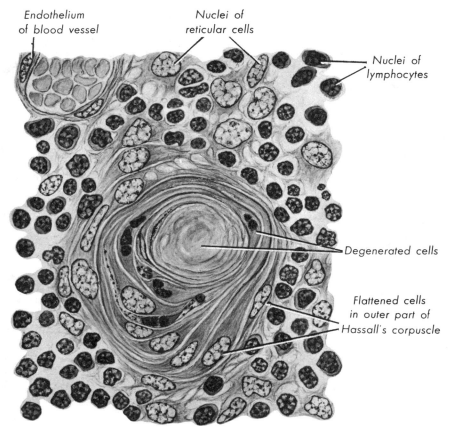

Figure 9.4. Diagram of the thymic medulla displaying Hassall's corpuscle. (From Copenhaver WM, Bunge RP, Bunge MB: *Bailey's Textbook of Histology*, ed. 16. Baltimore, Williams & Wilkins, 1971.)

gions of the lymph nodes and spleen. Mitotic activity of lymphocytes is much greater in the cortex of the thymus than in the medulla.

Spleen

—is the largest lymphatic organ in the body. Since it is an intraperitoneal organ, it is covered by a simple squamous epithelium (peritoneum).

—functions in filtering blood, storing erythrocytes, phagocytosing damaged and aged red blood cells, acting as a site of proliferation of B and T lymphocytes and the manufacture of antibodies.

—differs from the other lymphatic organs, in that it lacks a cortex and a medulla.

—is divided into regions designated as red pulp and white pulp.

Nerves, Blood, and Lymph Vessels

—enter and leave the spleen at its hilus, although the few (relatively small) afferent lymph vessels that the spleen possesses enter along its convex surface.

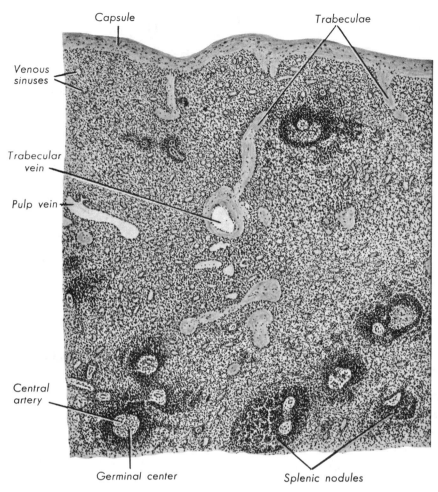

Figure 9.5. Diagram of a section of the spleen. (From Copenhaver WM, Bunge RP, Bunge MB: *Bailey's Textbook of Histology*, ed 16. Baltimore, Williams & Wilkins, 1971.)

Capsule
—is composed of dense, irregular collagenous connective tissue interspersed with elastic fibers and smooth muscle cells and is thicker at the hilus.

Trabeculae
—derived from the capsule convey blood vessels and nerves to and from the splenic pulp. Attached to the internal aspect of the capsule and trabeculae is a network of reticular fibers that forms the framework of the spleen.

Vascularization
—is derived from the splenic artery that enters the hilus, giving rise to trabecular arteries that are distributed to the splenic pulp via trabeculae.

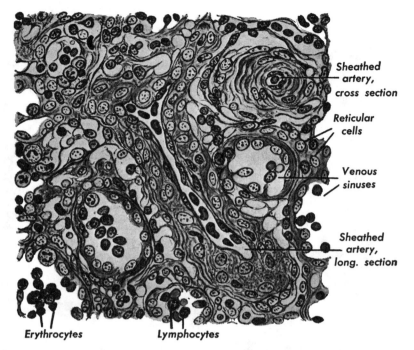

Figure 9.6. Diagram of the sheathed arterioles and venous sinuses of the spleen. (From Copenhaver WM, Bunge RP, Bunge MB: *Bailey's Textbook of Histology*, ed 16. Baltimore, Williams & Wilkins, 1971.)

—as these arteries leave the trabeculae they become invested by a sheath of lymphocytes and penetrate lymphatic nodules, where they are designated central arteries.

Central Arteries

—branch but maintain their lymphatic sheaths until they leave the white pulp to form several penicillar arteries.

Penicillar Arteries

—possess three regions: pulp arterioles, sheathed arterioles, and terminal arterial capillaries.

Terminal Arterial Capillaries

—either drain directly into the splenic sinusoids (closed circulation) or terminate as open-ended vessels within the red pulp (open circulation).

—splenic sinusoids are drained by pulp veins, which are branches of the trabecular veins, which in turn are tributaries of the splenic vein.

White Pulp

—is composed of all of the diffuse and nodular lymphoid tissue of the spleen.

—includes the central artery and the sheath of lymphocytes (periarterial lymphatic sheath, PALS) and lymphatic nodules (with occasional germinal centers) surrounding it.

—lymphatic nodules consist mainly of B lymphocytes.

—periarterial lymphatic sheaths are composed primarily of T lymphocytes.

—antigen-presenting cells and macrophages are also present in the white pulp.

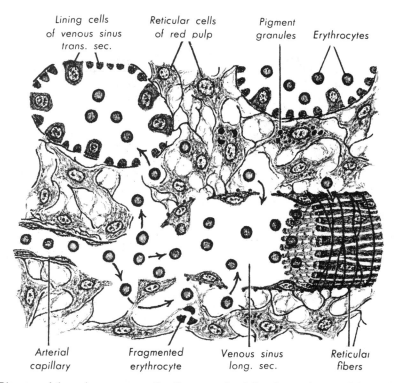

Figure 9.7. Diagram of the spleen, representing the open circulation theory. **Lower right**, three-dimensional representation of the venous sinus. Rib-like basement membrane associated with reticular fibers surrounds the elongated endothelial cells. (From Copenhaver WM, Kelly DE, Wood RL: *Bailey's Textbook of Histology*, ed 17. Baltimore, Williams & Wilkins, 1978.)

Marginal Zone

—is a region between the red and white pulps that receives capillary loops from the central artery, which drain into small sinusoids located at the periphery of the lymphatic nodules.

—is the first site where blood contacts the splenic parenchyma, and is richly supplied by avidly phagocytic macrophages and antigen-presenting cells.

—is the site where T and B lymphocytes enter the spleen prior to becoming segregated to their specific locations within the organ.

Red Pulp

—is composed of an interconnected network of sinusoids supported by a loose type of reticular tissue consisting of splenic cords (cords of Billroth).

Sinusoids

—are unusual in structure.

—their endothelial cells are long and fusiform, with relatively large intercellular spaces. Outside the endothelium are circumferentially arranged "ribs" composed of filamentous material and containing a few collagen fibrils.

—"ribs" appear to constitute a thick, discontinuous basal lamina supported by reticular fibers.

Splenic Cords

—contain plasma cells, reticular cells, various types of blood cells, and macrophages enmeshed within the spaces of the reticular fiber network.

—processes of the macrophages enter the lumina of the sinusoids through the large intercellular spaces between the sinusoidal lining cells.

REVIEW TESTS
LYMPHATIC TISSUE

DIRECTIONS: *One* or *more* of the given completions is/are correct. Choose answer:

    A. if only **1**, **2**, and **3** are correct
    B. if only **1** and **3** are correct
    C. if only **2** and **4** are correct
    D. if only **4** is correct
    E. if **all** are correct

9.1. T-helper cells
1. can assist only T lymphocytes
2. never assist B lymphocytes
3. are memory cells
4. produce lymphokines

9.2. Cytotoxic cells
1. kill foreign cells
2. may be a subgroup of T lymphocytes
3. may be natural killer cells
4. may be thymic-independent cells

9.3. The humoral response is suppressed by cells bearing
1. IgE receptors
2. IgM receptors
3. IgA receptors
4. IgG receptors

9.4. Interferon is
1. produced by T-helper cells
2. a substance that activates NK cells
3. a lymphokine
4. a substance that activates T-killer cells

9.5. Antibodies are produced by
1. T-memory cells
2. B-memory cells
3. T-helper cells
4. plasma cells

9.6. Epithelial reticular cells of the thymus
1. are found in the cortex
2. participate in the formation of the blood-thymus barrier
3. are derived from the third pharyngeal pouch
4. rest on basal laminae

9.7. Hassal's corpuscles
1. are found in the cortex of young individuals
2. are found in the cortex of old individuals
3. are derived from mesoderm
4. are found in the medulla of old individuals

9.8. The thymic-dependent zone of lymphocytes is in the
1. paracortex of the lymph node
2. cortical lymphatic nodules of the lymph node
3. periarterial lymphatic sheaths of the spleen
4. lymphatic nodules of the spleen

9.9. Unusual endothelial cells are found in the
1. cortex of the lymph node
2. paracortex of the lymph node
3. white pulp of the spleen
4. red pulp of the spleen

9.10. Numerous afferent lymphatics bearing valves are found in the
1. spleen
2. thymus
3. lymphatic nodules
4. lymph nodes

DIRECTIONS: The following questions or statements refer to the photomicrograph (Fig. 9.8). The letters on the figure are answers to the numbered items appearing below the photomicrograph. For each numbered item select the *one* letter that *best* corresponds to that item. Each letter may be used once, more than once, or not at all.

Figure 9.8. From Gartner LP, Hiatt JL: *Atlas of Histology*. Baltimore, Williams & Wilkins, 1987.

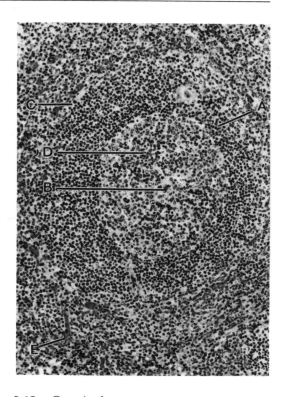

9.11. Central artery

9.12. Corona

9.13. Germinal center

9.14. Marginal zone

DIRECTIONS: The following questions or statements refer to the photomicrograph (Fig. 9.9). The letters on the figure are answers to the numbered items appearing below the photomicrograph. For each numbered item select the *one* letter that *best* corresponds to that item. Each letter may be used once, more than once, or not at all.

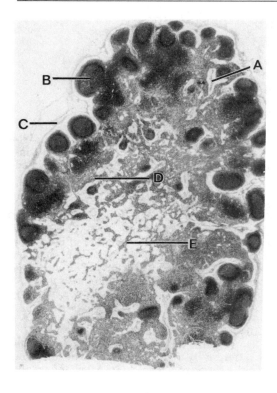

Figure 9.9. From Gartner LP, Hiatt JL: *Atlas of Histology*. Baltimore, Williams & Wilkins, 1987.

9.15. Trabecula

9.16. Medullary cord

9.17. Thymic-dependent zone

9.18. B-lymphocyte proliferation

ANSWERS AND EXPLANATIONS

LYMPHATIC TISSUE

9.1. D (4)

T-helper cells produce lymphokines and assist B-lymphocytes to combat thymic-dependent antigens. T-memory cells are a subgroup of T-lymphocytes, as are T-helper cells.

9.2. E (1,2,3, and 4)

The term *cytotoxic* refers to cells that kill other cells. T-killer cells and natural killer (NK) cells are both cytotoxic. Moreover, NK cells are thymic independent, in that they do not need to be potentiated by the thymus and can function even in athymic individuals.

9.3. D (4)

The humoral response is suppressed by T-suppressor cells that bear IgG receptors on their surface.

9.4. A (1,2, and 3)

Interferon is a lymphokine, produced by T-helper cells, that activates natural killer (NK) cells. It does not affect T-killer cells.

9.5. D (4)

Antibodies are produced by plasma cells. Neither memory cells nor T-helper cells possess the ability to synthesize antibodies.

9.6. E (1,2,3, and 4)

Epithelial reticular cells isolate the forming T-lymphocytes in the thymic cortex from all antigenic influences and thus assist in the formation of the blood-thymus barrier. Since they are epithelial cells (originating from the third pharyngeal pouch) they possess their own basal lamina.

9.7. D (4)

Hassal's (thymic) corpuscles are concentrically arranged epithelial reticular cells (derived from endoderm) found only in the medulla of the thymus. Their number increases with age.

9.8. B (1 and 3)

T lymphocytes are preferentially located in the paracortex of the lymph node and the periarterial lymphatic sheath of the spleen. B lymphocytes are found in lymphatic nodules located in the lymph node (cortex) and the spleen.

9.9. C (2 and 4)

Postcapillary venules of the lymph node paracortex possess cuboidal endothelial cells, and the sinusoids of the splenic red pulp possess spindle-shaped endothelial cells. Most other endothelial cells are attenuated simple squamous cells. The cortex of lymph nodes and the white pulp of the spleen have vessels lined by typical simple squamous endothelial cells.

9.10. D (4)

The thymus and lymphatic nodules receive no afferent lymphatic vessels. The afferent lymph vessels of the spleen are few and small. However, lymph nodes possess large, afferent lympatic channels, whose valves ensure a unidirectional flow of lymph through the node.

For questions **9.11** to **9.14**, refer to Figure 9.8.

9.11. B, Central artery.

9.12. A, Corona

9.13. D, Germinal center

9.14. C, Marginal zone

For questions **9.15** to **9.18**, refer to, Figure 9.9.

9.15. A, trabecula

9.16. E, medullary cord

9.17. D, thymic-dependent zone

9.18. B, B-lymphocyte proliferation

10
Endocrine System

Endocrine System

—is composed of several glands (pituitary, thyroid, parathyroid, suprarenal, and pineal body);
—clusters of cells located within certain organs (islets of Langerhans, interstitial cells of Leydig, etc.);
—individual cells distributed among the parenchymal cells in certain organs (APUD cells).

Endocrine Glands
—are discussed in this chapter. The other components are described in chapters discussing the organs in which they are located.
—produce hormones (chemical messengers) that enter the bloodstream to be carried to distant target organs.

Hormones
—are either low-molecular-weight proteins or lipid-soluble substances that activate parenchymal cells of the target organ by binding to specific receptor sites.
—receptors are located either on the external plasma membranes of the receptor cell (for proteins) or within the cytoplasm (for lipid-soluble hormones), which are then transported into the nucleus.

Components
—of the endocrine (and to a certain extent the nervous) system are interrelated in that they interact with and control each other's activities while they modulate and integrate the metabolic activities of the body.

Pituitary Gland

—Pituitary gland (hypophysis) is small (0.5 g) and is derived embryologically from the floor of the diencephalon and the roof of the pharynx (Rathke's pouch). This is reflected in its structure and function. This gland is composed of two major subdivisions, the adenohypophysis and the neurohypophysis.

Adenohypophysis
—is subdivided into the pars anterior (pars distalis), pars tuberalis (pars infundibularis), and the pars intermedia.

Neurohypophysis

—consists of the infundibular stalk and the pars nervosa. The pituitary gland maintains its connection with the hypothalamus via the infundibular stalk.

Vascular Supply

—of the pituitary gland arises from two pairs of vessels derived from the internal carotid artery.
—right and left superior hypophyseal arteries serve the median eminence, pars tuberalis, and infundibulum.
—right and left inferior hypophyseal arteries serve mostly the pars nervosa.

Branches

—of the superior hypophyseal arteries end in the primary capillary plexus within the substance of the median eminence and the base of the infundibulum.
—primary capillary plexus is drained by portal veins, which follow the infundibulum and enter the adenohypophysis where they form a secondary capillary plexus in the vicinity of the parenchymal cells.

Hormones (factors)

—released by neurosecretory cells of the median eminence are able to modulate the activity of the parenchymal cells of the adenohypophysis via this hypophyseal portal system.

Adenohypophysis
Pars Anterior

Architecture

—consists of a collagenous capsule surrounding cords of parenchymal cells that are irregularly arranged among large sinusoids. The glandular cells and the vasculature deep within the gland are supported by reticular fibers.

Parenchymal Cells

—are of two major types, chromophils, which possess a strong affinity for histologic stains, and chromophobes, cells whose granules do not readily take up stains.

Chromophils

—are of two types, the acidophils, which stain pink, and the basophils, which stain blue. "Acidic" and "basic" in this context is in relationship to the secretory granules rather than to the cytoplasm of the cells.

Acidophils

—are usually located in the center and posterolateral regions of the pars anterior.
—are small, spherical cells (15 to 20 μm diameter) that are of two subtypes, somatotrophs and mammotrophs.

Somatotrophs

—produce the hormone somatotropin [growth hormone (GH)], which is contained within spherical, membrane-bounded granules (300 to 400 nm diameter) in the cells.
—possess a centrally positioned nucleus, moderate-sized Golgi apparatus, rod-shaped mitochondria, and abundant rough endoplasmic reticulum.

Mammotrophs

—produce the hormone prolactin, which they store in small (200 nm) membrane-bounded granules.

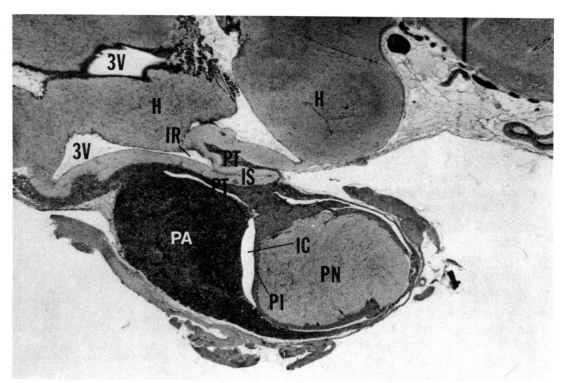

Figure 10.1. Photomicrograph of the pituitary gland demonstrating its relationship to the hypothalamus: **H**, hypothalamus; **3V**, third ventricle; **PT**, pars tuberalis; **IS**, infundibular stem; **IR**, infundibular process; **PA**, pars anterior; **IC**, intraglandular cleft; **PI**, pars intermedia; **PN**, nervosa. × 19. (From Gartner LP, Hiatt JL: *Atlas of Histology*. Baltimore, Williams & Wilkins, 1987.)

—secretory granules become enlarged (to 600 nm diameter) in pregnant and lactating women, and the organelle population increases.

—granules remaining in mammotrophs after suckling are destroyed by lysosomal enzymes. This process, involving autophagic vacuoles, is known as crinophagy.

Basophils
—stain more intensely than acidophils and are usually located at the periphery of the pars anterior. There are three subtypes of basophils: corticotrophs, thyrotrophs, and gonadotrophs.

Corticotrophs
—produce adrenocorticotropic (ACTH) and lipotropic (LPH, a β-endorphin precursor) hormones that are stored in small (200 to 250 nm diameter) granules.

—are spherical to ovoid-shaped cells whose cytoplasm displays relatively few organelles and an acentric nucleus. Occasionally corticotrophs are present in the pars nervosa.

Thyrotrophs
—produce thyroid-stimulating hormone (TSH) that is stored in small (150 nm diameter) secretory granules that are often located just beneath the cell membrane.

Gonadotrophs
—produce follicle-stimulating hormone (FSH) and luteinizing hormone (LH) that are stored in granules whose diameters vary from 200 to 400 nm.

—are well endowed with rough endoplasmic reticulum and mitochondria and have a well-developed Golgi apparatus.

Chromophobes
—probably represent several cell types.

—light micrographs demonstrate that these small cells appear to lack secretory granules and that they are arranged as clusters whose nuclei are close to one another.

—electron micrographs demonstrate that some of these cells resemble degranulated chromophils, suggesting that they represent different stages in the life cycle of various acidophil and basophil populations.

—additionally some chromophobes may belong to a group of undifferentiated regenerative cells that are capable of differentiating into various types of chromophils.

Folliculostellate Cells
—are nongranular, with long processes that are also present in the pars distalis.

—may support the parenchymal cells, although it has been suggested that they may be phagocytic.

Hormones of the Pars Anterior
Somatotropin (GH)
—produced by the acidophils (somatotrophs), is a linear protein molecule (MW 21,500).

—functions to increase the metabolic rate of most cells. In young individuals it indirectly (via somatomedin intermediaries) increases the proliferative activity of the epiphyseal plates of long bones.

Prolactin
—produced by the acidophils (mammotrophs), is a linear protein molecule (MW 25,000) that facilitates the maturation of the mammary gland during pregnancy and lactation.

Adrenocorticotropic Hormone (ACTH)

—produced by the basophils (corticotrophs), is a small (MW 4,500) linear protein molecule cleaved from the larger molecule pro-opiocortin.

—functions to stimulate cells of the zona glomerulosa of the suprarenal gland to manufacture and release cortisol.

—β-lipotropic hormone is a second cleavage product derived from pro-opiocortin that has no known function (although it may be further cleaved into melanocyte-stimulating hormone and β-endorphin.

Thyroid-Stimulating Hormone (TSH)

—produced by the basophils (thyrotrophs), is a glycoprotein (MW 28,000) that stimulates the thyroid gland to synthesize and release thyroxine (T_4) and triiodothyronine (T_3).

Follicle-Stimulating Hormone (FSH)

—produced by the basophils (gonadotrophs), is a glycoprotein (MW 30,000).

—in females it is responsible for the cyclic maturation of ovarian follicles.

—in males it facilitates spermatogenesis (by stimulating Sertoli cells to produce androgen-binding protein).

Luteinizing Hormone (LH)

—produced by the same basophils (gonadotrophs) that manufacture FSH.

—is a glycoprotein (MW 28,000).

—in females it induces ovulation and is involved in the transformation of the remnants of the graafian follicle into the corpus luteum.

—in males it is also known as interstitial cell-stimulating hormone (ICSH), and it acts on the interstitial cells of Leydig to secrete testosterone.

Hormonal Control Systems

Specific Neurosecretory Cells

—of the hypothalamus, subsequent to becoming activated, cause the release of hypophyseotropic hormones (releasing factors), which enter the hypophyseal portal system to stimulate or inhibit the parenchymal cells of the adenohypophysis.

—they are in turn regulated by hormonal blood levels (negative feedback).

Thyrotropin-Releasing Hormone (TRH)

—is a tripeptide that facilitates the release of TSH from the adenohypophysis.

Corticotropin-Releasing Hormone (CRH)

—is a small protein that induces the release of ACTH.

Gonadotropin-Releasing Hormone (GnRH)

—a small peptide that triggers the release of FSH and LH.

Prolactin-Releasing Hormone (PRH)

—has not been characterized biochemically, but it is believed to facilitate the release of prolactin.

Dopamine

—a precursor of catecholamines, inhibits the release of prolactin.

Somatostatin

—a polypeptide composed of 14 amino acids, inhibits the release of growth hormone.

Pars Intermedia

—is small in the human.

—characterized by the presence of numerous colloid-containing cysts (Rathke's cysts) lined by ciliated cuboidal cells.

—Rathke's cysts are remnants of the cleft that separates the adeno- and neurohypophysis in some animals.

—cells of the pars intermedia are basophils (which project into the substance of the neurohypophysis). They secrete melanocyte-stimulating hormone (MSH).

Pars Tuberalis

—in the human is small.

—composed of cords of cuboidal cells, some cuboidal cell–lined follicles, a few basophils, and an extremely rich vascular supply (composed of the superior hypophyseal arteries and hypophyseal venous portal system).

—basophils secrete FSH and LH.

Neurohypophysis

—composed of the pars nervosa and the infundibular stalk.

—resembles nervous tissue and is composed of unmyelinated axons of neurosecretory cells whose soma are located in the supraoptic and paraventricular nuclei (of the median eminence) in the hypothalamus.

Figure 10.2. Diagram of the hypothalamohypophyseal tract. (From Copenhaver WM, Bunge RP, Bunge MB: *Bailey's Textbook of Histology*, ed 16. Baltimore, Williams & Wilkins, 1971.)

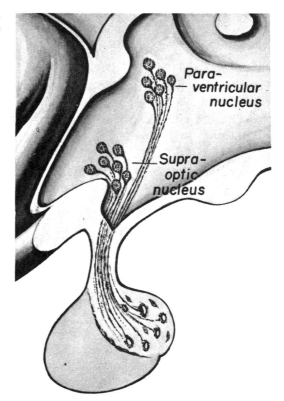

Axons

—of these cells represent the hypothalamohypophyseal tract, and they are supported by pituicytes (glial-like cells).

—display swellings, known as Herring bodies, containing neurosecretory material along their lengths and at their blind ends.

Herring Bodies

—are filled with vesicles containing neurosecretion (oxytocin and vasopressin).

—neurosecretions (upon stimulation) are released from the ends of the axons in the vicinity of fenestrated capillaries (derived from the inferior hypophyseal arteries).

Oxytocin

—is one of the hormones released by neurosecretory axons in the neurohypophysis.

—induces smooth muscle contraction, including that in the wall of the uterus (during copulation and parturition), as well as contraction of myoepithelial cells of the mammary gland (during nursing).

Vasopressin (Antidiuretic Hormone; ADH)

—is a hormone released in the neurohypophysis by axons of the neurosecretory cells.

—functions to render the walls of the renal collecting tubules permeable to water, which is absorbed, producing a concentrated urine.

—also functions as a vasoconstrictor of smooth cells in the tunica media of arterioles.

Neurophysins

—are released along with oxytocin and vasopressin. They are believed to be binding proteins (one for each hormone) whose precise functions are not known.

Pituicytes

—have numerous processes. They resemble neuroglial cells and contain lipid droplets, intermediate filaments, and pigments.

Thyroid Gland

—is composed of two lobes connected by an isthmus. It is located in the anterior triangle of the neck, slightly below the level of the cricoid cartilage.

Capsule

—is composed of a dense outer connective tissue layer in which the parathyroid glands are embedded and a loose inner connective tissue layer.

—septa derived from the inner layer, not only serve as conduits for blood vessels but also subdivide the gland into incomplete lobules containing follicles.

Follicles

—consist of spherical colloid-filled structures lined by simple cuboidal epithelial cells (which constitute the parenchyma of the thyroid gland).

—cells are of two types, follicular and parafollicular cells, comprising the epithelium, which is enveloped by a basal lamina that separates it from the surrounding rich vascular supply and connective tissue.

Follicular Cells

—are usually cuboidal and constitute the majority of the cells lining the follicle.

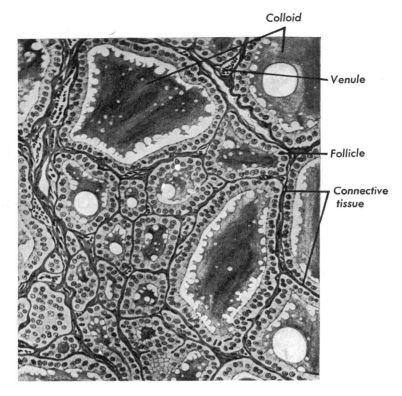

Figure 10.3. Diagram of the adult human thyroid gland. (From Copenhaver WM, Kelly DE, Wood RL: *Bailey's Textbook of Histology*, ed 17. Baltimore, Williams & Wilkins, 1978.)

—border the colloid (a viscous gel consisting mostly of iodinated thyroglobulin) contained with the follicle.

—can become columnar when they are actively secreting and are being stimulated, but in the resting state they appear low cuboidal.

—produce the glycoprotein thyroglobulin, which serves as the storage site for the two thyroid hormones (T_3 and T_4) also produced by these cells. T_3 and T_4, upon stimulation by TSH, are released basally into the bloodstream and circulate to many organs, producing an increase in the basal metabolic rate.

—possess short, blunt microvilli in the normal gland but form pseudopods that engulf large amounts of colloid when stimulated by TSH.

Organelles

—rough endoplasmic reticulum, supranuclear Golgi apparatus, and few, rod-shaped mitochondria.

Apical Vesicles

—are associated with the release of thyroglobulin into the colloid.

—reverse transit occurs when TSH stimulates the uptake of colloid droplets, their fusion with lysosomes, and the controlled hydrolysis that releases T_3 and T_4 basally into the vascular system.

Parafollicular Cells (clear cells)

—produce calcitonin (thyrocalcitonin) (MW 3,500), a hormone that lowers blood calcium levels.
—do not contact the colloid and are located individually or in small clusters between the follicular cells and basal lamina (within the follicle).
—are recognizable histologically as clear cells, since they do not stain as intensely as the follicular cells.
—electron micrographs demonstrate that these cells contain elongated mitochondria, a substantial amount of rough endoplasmic reticulum, a well-developed Golgi apparatus, and numerous membrane-bounded secretory granules (100 to 300 nm diameter), which represent calcitonin.

Parathyroid Glands

—are four in number and lie embedded in the thyroid capsule (on its posterior surface).
—parenchyma is composed of two types of cells, chief cells and oxyphils (although an intermediate cell type has also been described).
—in older individuals become infiltrated with fat cells.

Capsule

—is composed of slender collagenous connective tissue strands.
—septa, derived from the capsule, penetrate the substance of the gland to support the parenchymal elements and to convey blood vessels into the interior of the gland.

Chief Cells

—synthesize and secrete parathyroid hormone (MW 9,500), which is responsible for maintaining proper levels of blood calcium and phosphate.
—are small, polyhedral in shape, and clustered to form anastomosing cords, which are surrounded by a rich vascular supply.
—electron micrographs reveal the presence of a centrally placed, spherical nucleus, a well-developed Golgi apparatus, abundant rough endoplasmic reticulum, small mitochondria, glycogen deposits, and numerous variable-shaped secretory granules (0.2 to 0.4 μm diameter).

Oxyphil Cells

—are large, eosinophilic cells that form small clusters within the parenchyma of the gland.
—function is unknown, but they increase in number with age.
—electron micrographs reveal a cytoplasm literally filled with elongated mitochondria. The remaining dense cytoplasm has a poorly developed Golgi apparatus and only a limited amount of rough endoplasmic reticulum.

Suprarenal Glands

—Suprarenal glands (adrenal glands) lie embedded in fat at the superior poles of the kidneys and are invested in their own connective tissue capsule.
—are derived from two separate embryonic sources: neural crest (giving rise to the medulla), and mesodermal epithelium (the source for the cortex).
—septa, derived from the dense irregular collagenous capsule, penetrate the substance of the gland, conveying a rich vascular supply.

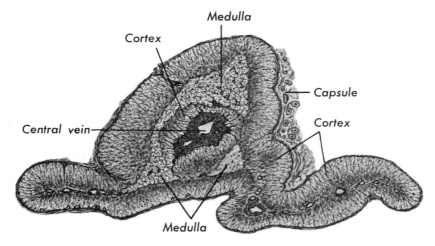

Figure 10.4. Drawing of a section of the human suprarenal gland. (From Kelly DE, Wood RL, Enders AC: *Bailey's Textbook of Microscopic Anatomy*, ed 18. Baltimore, Williams & Wilkins, 1984.)

Cortex

Suprarenal Cortex

—is subdivided into three concentric, histologically recognizable regions: the zona glomerulosa, zona fasciculata, and zona reticularis.

Zona Glomerulosa

—is located just beneath the capsule and is the thinnest layer of the cortex.

—is composed of parenchymal cells arranged in arch-like cords and round clusters.

Parenchymal Cells

—are acidophilic and are smaller than those of the zona fasciculata.

—possess only a few small lipid droplets and have dense, round nuclei containing one or two nucleoli.

—electron micrographs demonstrate that the cells contain an extensive network of smooth endoplasmic reticulum, short mitochondria, a well-developed Golgi apparatus, rough endoplasmic reticulum, and free ribosomes.

—function in producing mineralocorticoids, namely aldosterone and deoxycorticosterone.

Aldosterone Release

—is triggered by angiotensin II (as well as ACTH), and it stimulates the resorption of sodium and the excretion of potassium by distal tubules of the kidney.

Zona Fasciculata

—occupies the largest area of the cortex (up to 80%).

—cells are large, polyhedral (spongiocytes) and are filled with lipid droplets.

—are arranged, one to two layers thick, in longitudinal columns that are oriented perpendicularly to the capsule. Extending between neighboring columns are longitudinally oriented sinusoidal capillaries.

—electron micrographs of spongiocytes display a considerable network of smooth endoplasmic reticulum, a large Golgi apparatus, some rough endoplasmic reticulum, and numerous large, cylindrical mitochondria. Lysosomes and lipochrome pigment are also present.

—lipid droplets are also evident, but they are more numerous in the peripheral region of the zona fasciculata (near the zona glomerulosa) than in its deeper aspect.

—function to produce and release (in response to ACTH) androgens (dehydroepiandrosterone) and glucocorticoids (corticosterone and cortisol).

Zona Reticularis

—is the deepest layer of the cortex, whose parenchymal cells are arranged in anastomosing cords.

Parenchymal Cells

—are smaller in size and possess fewer lipid granules than cells of the zona fasciculata.

—some cells display pyknotic nuclei and have many lipofuscin pigment inclusions. Some authors suggest that there are two populations of cells, dark (degenerative) and light (functional) cells.

—function is to manufacture and release (under the influence of ACTH) androgens (dehydroepiandrosterone) and perhaps glucocorticoids (corticosterone and cortisol).

Medulla

Suprarenal Medulla

—is completely invested by the cortex.

Parenchymal Cells

—are arranged in short, irregular cords and are surrounded by an extremely rich capillary network.

—are innervated by preganglionic sympathetic fibers and are considered to serve the function of postganglionic sympathetic neurons.

—synthesize and release epinephrine and norepinephrine.

—are of three different types: two populations of chromaffin cells and a few large postganglionic sympathetic nerve cell bodies.

Chromaffin Cells

—are large, polyhedral cells whose granules (chromaffin granules) stain intensely with chromiun salts (chromaffin reaction).

—morphologically the two populations of cells are identical. They may be distinguished from one another by special staining techniques because they produce different catecholamines (epinephrine and norepinephrine).

—light micrographs demonstrate that these cells possess an epithelioid appearance, have a pale cytoplasm containing chromaffin granules, and often display large, vesicular nuclei with a single, large nucleolus.

—electron micrographs exhibit a well-developed Golgi apparatus, isolated regions of rough endoplasmic reticulum, numerous mitochondria, and large numbers of membrane-bounded secretory granules (0.1 to 0.3 μm diameter).

—granule size permits differentiation of the two populations of chromaffin cells.

—epinephrine-producing cells possess homogeneous granules.

—norepinephrine-producing cells have an extremely electron-dense center with a peripheral electron-lucent halo beneath their membranous envelope.

—catecholamine release is stimulated by the preganglionic parasympathetic fiber innervating the medulla. The chromaffin granules also contain ATP, enkephalins, and chromogranins.

Pineal Body

Pineal Body (epiphysis)

—a flat, small projection of the roof of the diencephalon.

—capsule is formed by the pia mater, from which septa and trabeculae extend to subdivide the pineal body into incomplete lobules.

—trabeculae derived from the capsule convey vascular elements into the interior of the gland.

Cellular Elements

—pinealocytes and neuroglial cells.

Interstitium

—contains calcified accretions of unknown function, known as brain sand (corpora arenacea, acervuli).

Pinealocytes

—are pale-staining cells that possess numerous long processes that end in bulb-like dilatations in the vicinity of capillaries.

—possess large nuclei, a well-developed smooth endoplasmic reticulum, some rough endoplasmic reticulum, free ribosomes, a Golgi apparatus, and numerous secretory granules.

—also possess microtubules and microfilaments, as well as unusual structures (syn-

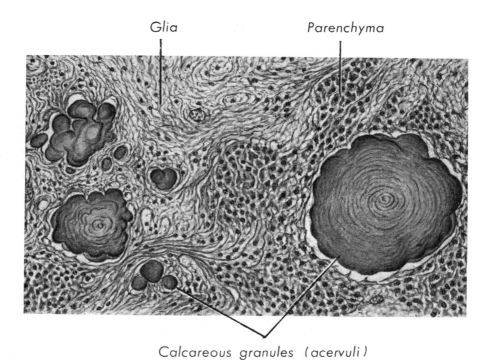

Glia   Parenchyma

Calcareous granules (acervuli)

Figure 10.5. Drawing of a section of the human pineal body displaying acervuli. (From Kelly DE, Wood RL, Enders AC: *Bailey's Textbook of Microscopic Anatomy*, ed 18. Baltimore, Williams & Wilkins, 1984.)

aptic ribbons) composed of dense tubular elements surrounded by synaptic vesicle-like spheroids whose function remains unclear.

—function in producing serotonin (usually during the day) and melatonin (usually at night). They may also produce arginine vasotocin, a peptide that might be an antagonist of LH and FSH.

Neuroglial Cells (interstitial cells)

—resemble astrocytes, with elongated processes and small, densely stained, oval nuclei.

—electron micrographs reveal the presence of rough endoplasmic reticulum, microtubules, many microfilaments (7 nm diameter), and intermediate filaments (10 nm diameter).

REVIEW TESTS

ENDOCRINE SYSTEM

DIRECTIONS: *One* or *more* of the given statements or completions is/are correct. Choose answer:

    A. if only **1**, **2**, and **3** are correct
    B. if only **1** and **3** are correct
    C. if only **2** and **4** are correct
    D. if only **4** is correct
    E. if **all** are correct

10.1. Hormones that are protein in nature exert their effects by
1. attaching to receptors on the nuclear membrane
2. attaching to receptors in the nucleolus
3. diffusing through the plasma membrane
4. attaching to receptors on the plasma membrane

10.2. Chromaffin cells
1. of the zona fasciculata produce androgens
2. of the suprarenal medulla produce epinephrine
3. of the zona glomerulosa produce mineralocorticoids
4. contain catecholamines

10.3. Pinealocytes of the pineal body
1. produce melatonin
2. are astrocyte-like cells
3. produce serotonin
4. are postganglionic sympathetic soma

10.4. The thyroid follicles
1. contain thyroglobulin
2. are usually lined by a simple cuboidal epithelium
3. contain follicular cells that release thyroxin
4. contain parafollicular cells that release calcitonin

10.5. Oxyphil cells are present in the
1. adenohypophysis
2. pineal gland
3. neurohypophysis
4. parathyroid gland

10.6. Melanocyte-stimulating hormone (MSH) is produced by
1. acidophils of the pars nervosa
2. basophils of the pars anterior
3. acidophils of the pars intermedia
4. basophils of the pars intermedia

10.7. Adrenocorticotropic hormone (ACTH) is produced by
1. basophils of the pars anterior
2. neurosecretory cells in the median eminence
3. corticotrophs of the adenohypophysis
4. cells of the paraventricular nucleus in the hypothalamus

DIRECTIONS: The following questions or statements refer to the photomicrographs (Figs. 10.6 and 10.7). The letters on the figures are answers to the numbered items appearing below the photomicrographs. For each numbered item, select the *one* letter that *best* corresponds to that item. Each letter may be used once, more than once, or not at all.

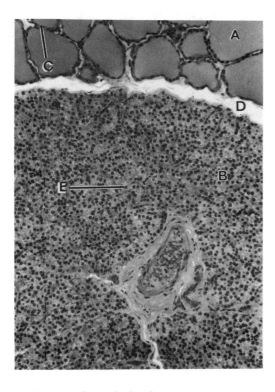

Figure 10.6. From Gartner LP, Hiatt JL: *Atlas of Histology.* Baltimore, Williams & Wilkins, 1987.

10.8. parathyroid gland

10.9. colloid

10.10. follicular cell

10.11. capsule

Figure 10.7. From Gartner LP, Hiatt JL: *Atlas of Histology*. Baltimore, Williams & Wilkins, 1987.

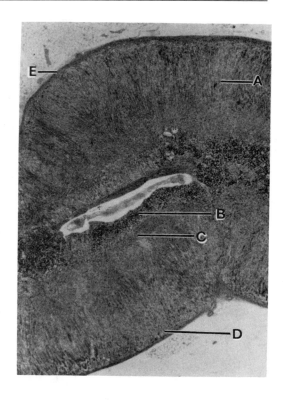

10.12. medulla

10.13. zona fasciculata

10.14. aldosterone release

10.15. location of postganglionic parasympathetic cell bodies

10.16. zona glomerulosa

10.17. zona reticularis

ANSWERS AND EXPLANATIONS

ENDOCRINE SYSTEM

10.1. D (4)

Hormones that are protein cannot diffuse through the cell membrane but attach to receptors on the external aspect of the plasmalemma.

10.2. C (2 and 4)

Chromaffin cells are located in the suprarenal medulla. They contain chromaffin granules, which represent epinephrine, norepinephrine, ATP, chromogranins, and enkephalins.

10.3. B (1 and 3)

The pineal body has two main cell types, pinealocytes and neuroglial cells. The pinealocytes produce and release melatonin and serotonin. There are no postganglionic sympathetic soma in the pineal.

10.4. E (1, 2, 3 and 4)

All of the statements are correct.

10.5. D (4)

Oxyphils are present only in the parathyroid gland. The adenohypophysis contains acidophils, the neurohypophysis possesses pituicytes, and the pineal gland has pinealocytes and neuroglial cells.

10.6. D (4)

Neither the pars nervosa nor the pars anterior produce melanocyte-stimulating hormone (MSH). Acidophils are not found in the pars intermedia, but basophils in this area produce MSH.

10.7. B (1 and 3)

Neurosecretory cells in the median eminence and the paraventricular cells in the hypothalamus produce hormones that control the release of hormones by the anterior pituitary. Adrenocorticotropic hormone (ACTH) is produced by corticotrophs (a type of basophil) present in the pars anterior of the adenohypophysis.

For questions **10.8** through **10.11**, refer to Figure **10.6**, a section of the thyroid and parathyroid gland.

10.8. B, parathyroid gland

10.9. A, colloid

10.10. C, follicular cell

10.11. D, capsule

For questions **10.12** through **10.17**, refer to Figure **10.7**, a section of the suprarenal gland.

10.12. B, medulla

10.13. A, zona fasciculata

10.14. D, aldosterone release

10.15. B, location of postganglionic parasympathetic cell bodies

10.16. D, zona glomerulosa

10.17. C, zona reticularis

11
Integument

Integument

—refers to the skin plus its appendages.

Skin

—covers the surface of the body and is composed of two layers, epidermis and dermis. The deeper fascial layer, the hypodermis, is not considered part of skin.
—serves several important functions: protection against injury, dessication, and infection; the regulation of body temperature; the absorption of UV radiation for synthesis of vitamin D; and the reception of sensory stimuli (tactile, thermal, and pain) from the external environment.
—epidermis and dermis interdigitate with each other to form an irregular contour. Dermal papillae (ridges) project into the epidermis to produce epidermal ridges (which can be seen on the finger tips with the naked eye).
—may also be classified as thick or thin, depending on the thickness of the epidermis.

Appendages of Skin

—include sweat glands, hair follicles, sebaceous glands, and nails.

General Structural Plan of Skin

Epidermis

Characteristics

—a stratified squamous keratinized epithelium, composed of several strata, which forms the superficial layer of skin.
—is constantly being regenerated by its keratinocytes (every 2 to 4 weeks) via mitotic activity that occurs mostly at night.
—epithelial layers of the epidermis include the following strata: basale, spinosum, granulosum, lucidum, and corneum.

Stratum Basale (germinativum)

—is the deepest layer of cells, attached directly to the basal lamina by hemidesmosomes.
—cuboidal to columnar in shape and frequently seen undergoing division.
—melanocytes (pigment cells) and Merkel cells are also present in this layer.

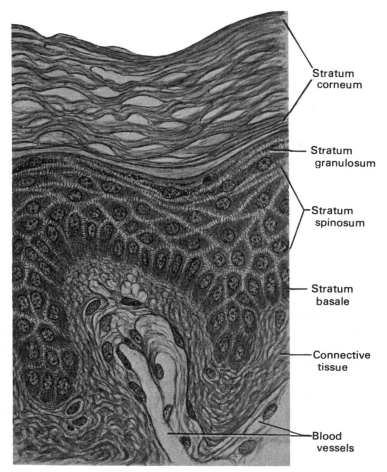

Figure 11.1. Drawing of a section of skin. (From Kelly DE, Wood RL, Enders AC: *Bailey's Textbook of Microscopic Anatomy*, ed 18. Baltimore, Williams & Wilkins, 1984.)

Stratum Spinosum

—consists of a few layers of polyhedral (prickle) keratinocytes.

—these cells have extensions, or so-called "intercellular bridges," where desmosomes attach the cells to each other.

—cells of this layer are mitotically active.

—in upper regions of the stratum spinosum are keratinocytes that contain membrane-coating granules, which are released into the intercellular spaces and cement the cells together, "waterproofing" the skin.

—Langerhans cells also present in this layer.

Stratum Malpighii

—refers to the stratum basale and the stratum spinosum grouped together.

Stratum Granulosum

—the layer of the epidermis where cells accumulate keratohyalin granules and bundles of intermediate keratin filaments (tonofilaments) and become flattened.

—also produce membrane-coating granules.

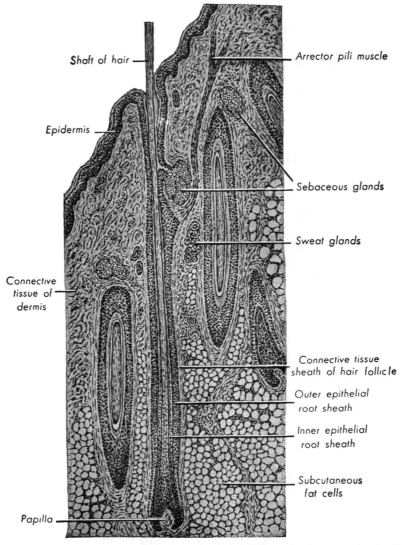

Figure 11.2. Drawing of a section of thin skin displaying hair follicles and sebaceous glands. (From Kelly DE, Wood RL, Enders AC: *Bailey's Textbook of Microscopic Anatomy*, ed 18. Baltimore, Williams & Wilkins, 1984.)

Keratohyalin Granules
—are not enclosed in a membrane but are composed of histidine- and cystine-rich proteins that appear to bind the keratin filaments together.

Cytoplasmic Aspect
—of the plasmalemma of these keratinocytes is thickened by an electron-dense layer, 10 to 12 nm thick, that reinforces it.

—is the most superficial layer in which nuclei are present.

Stratum Lucidum
—a clear homogeneous layer, which is often difficult to distinguish in histological sections.

—nuclei and organelles are not present in this layer, and the cells contain a substance known as eleidin, which is believed to be a transformation product of keratohyalin.

Stratum Corneum

—is the outermost layer of the epidermis.
—is composed of scale-like dead cells (squames).
—each squame is a 14-sided polygon.
—surface layers of cells are constantly being desquamated.
—region being desquamated is sometimes referred to as the stratum disjunctum.

Other Cell Types in the Epidermis

Melanocytes

—are present in the stratum basale and derived from the neural crest.
—synthesize brown melanin pigment in oval organelles called melanosomes.
—contain tyrosinase, a UV-sensitive enzyme directly involved in melanin synthesis.
—contain long processes that extend between the cells of the stratum spinosum.
—by way of these processes, the melanocytes transfer (or inject) melanosomes into keratinocytes in the stratum spinosum.
—this unique mechanism for the transfer of pigment is known as cytocrine secretion.
—once melanosomes are within the keratinocytes, they are degraded by lysosomes.
—number of melanocytes per unit area of skin varies from one part of the body to another but is independent of race.

Langerhans Cells

—are dendritic-shaped cells derived from the bone marrow.
—are present mainly in the stratum spinosum.
—contain distinct paddle-shaped membrane-bounded granules (Birbeck granules).
—function in presenting antigen to lymphocytes and thereby play a role in contact allergic responses.

Merkel Cells

—are present in small numbers in the stratum basale, near areas of connective tissue containing blood vessels and nerves.
—contain small dense-cored granules that are similar in appearance to those in cells of the adrenal medulla.
—receive afferent nerve terminals and are believed to function as sensory mechano-receptors.

Dermis (Corium)

Characteristics

—layer of skin underlying the epidermis that consists of dense, irregular connective tissue.
—contains collagen (Type I) fibers in abundance and networks of thick elastic fibers.
—is divided into a superficial papillary layer and a deeper more extensive reticular layer, but there is no distinct boundary between them.

Papillary Layer

—is uneven and forms dermal papillae that interdigitate with the basal surface of the epidermis.

—is composed of thin, loosely arranged fibers and cells.

—Meissner's corpuscles (fine-touch receptors) and capillary loops are located in this layer.

Reticular Layer

—forms the major portion of the dermis and contains thick, dense, irregular arrays of collagen fiber bundles and thick elastic fibers.

Encapsulated Nerve Endings

—consisting of Pacinian corpuscles (pressure receptors) and Krause's end bulbs (cold and pressure receptors) may be present in the deeper regions of the dermis.

Arrector Pili Muscle

—are bundles of smooth muscle, attached to hair follicles in the dermis, extend superficially to underlie sebaceous glands, and insert into the papillary layer of the dermis.

—contraction of arrector pili muscle elevates the hair and produces "goose bumps."

—deep to the reticular layer is the superficial fascia, or hypodermis, a loose connective tissue, containing many fat cells, that is not considered part of the skin.

Two Types of Skin

Thick Skin

—has a thick epidermis that is characterized by a prominent stratum corneum.

—lines the palms of the hands and the soles of the feet.

—*lacks* hair follicles, sebaceous glands, and arrector pili muscle bundles.

Thin Skin

—has a thin epidermis with a less prominent stratum corneum.

—is present over most of the body surface and contains hair follicles, sebaceous glands, and arrector pili muscle bundles.

—stratum lucidum and stratum granulosum are seldom seen in thin skin, although individual cells are present that show characteristics of these layers.

Glands

Eccrine Sweat Glands

—are distributed in skin throughout the body.

—are simple tubular coiled glands that have a secretory unit composed of three cell types: dark cells, clear cells, and myoepithelial cells.

Secretory Unit (of eccrine gland)

Dark Cells

—line the lumen and contain secretory granules.

Clear Cells

—underlie the dark cells and are rich in mitochondria and glycogen.

—passes intercellular canaliculi, which extend to the lumen of the secretory unit.

Myoepithelial Cells

—lie on the basal lamina, scattered beneath the clear cells.

Duct of Eccrine Gland

—is narrow and lined by a stratified cuboidal epithelium.

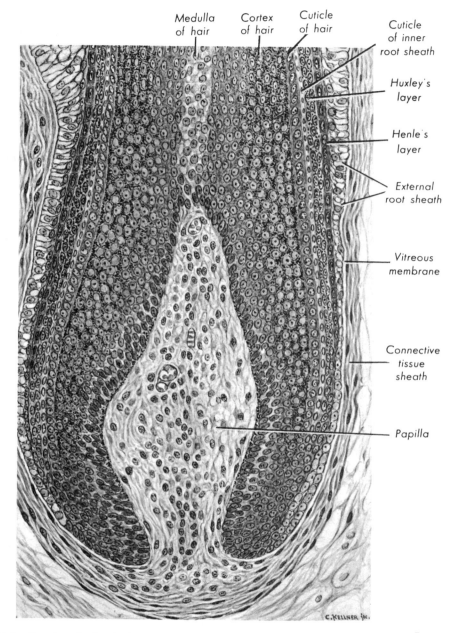

Figure 11.3. Drawing of a longitudinal section of the root of a hair follicle. (From Kelly DE, Wood RL, Enders AC: *Bailey's Textbook of Microscopic Anatomy*, ed 18. Baltimore, Williams & Wilkins, 1984.)

—leads from the secretory unit, through the superficial portions of the dermis, to penetrate the interpapillary peg of the epidermis and spiral through its layers to deliver sweat to the outside.

—cell type lining the narrow lumen of the sweat duct contains many keratin filaments and has a prominent terminal web.

—in contrast, the basal layer of cells has many mitochondria and prominent nuclei.

Apocrine Glands

—are large specialized sweat glands located in various areas of the body, such as the axilla, the areola of the nipple, and the circumanal region.

—do not begin to function until puberty and are responsive to hormonal influences.

—have a large coiled secretory portion enveloped by scattered myoepithelial cells.

—empty their viscous secretory products into hair follicles at a location superficial to the entry of ducts from sebaceous glands.

—are innervated by adrenergic fibers.

—*apocrine* implies that a portion of the cytoplasm becomes part of the secretion, but electron micrographs have shown that this is not true.

Ceruminous (wax) Glands

—of the external auditory canal are also included in this category.

Sebaceous Glands

—consist of several sacs (alveoli) that empty into a short duct, which in turn empties into the neck of a hair follicle.

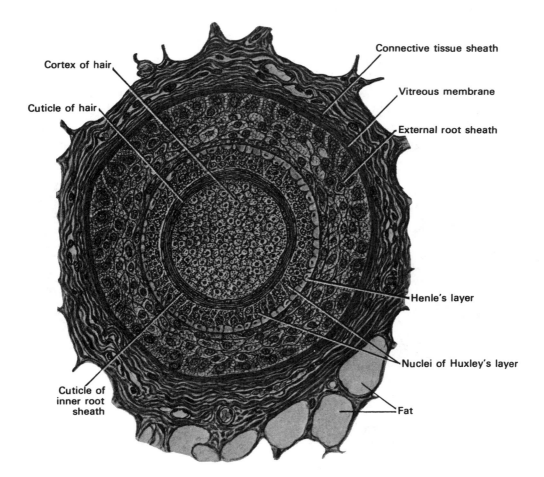

Figure 11.4. Drawing of a cross section of a hair follicle. (From Kelly DE, Wood RL, Enders AC: *Bailey's Textbook of Microscopic Anatomy*, ed 18. Baltimore, Williams & Wilkins, 1984.)

—cells at the periphery of the alveoli are flattened and inactive, but near the ducts mitoses are common.

—daughter cells migrate to the alveolus, produce a secretory product, and begin to break down, releasing an oily secretion known as sebum.

—process is known as holocrine secretion (both the disintegrated cells and the secretory material are discharged).

Hair Follicle

—a tubular invagination of the epidermis extending deep into the dermis.

—shaft of the hair projects above the surface of the epidermis.

—hair consists of a medulla, cortex, and cuticle.

—root of the hair is embedded in an expanded hair bulb, which is deeply indented by a papilla (of dermis).

—cells in the hair bulb form the inner epithelial root sheath and the medulla.

—internal root sheath is an epithelial structure (lying deep to the entrance of the sebaceous gland) composed of Henle's layer, Huxley's layer, and the cuticle.

—outer root sheath is a direct continuation of the stratum Malpighii of the epidermis.

—the next superficial layer is the glassy (basement) membrane, and the outermost layer is the connective tissue sheath (dermis).

Nail

—is located on the distal phalanx of each finger or toe.

—is composed of hard keratin lying on a nail bed.

—eponychium (cuticle) overlies the crescent-shaped whitish lunula.

—hyponychium (keratinized epithelial layer) is located beneath the free edge.

—cells in the nail matrix, at the root, are responsible for the growth of the nail.

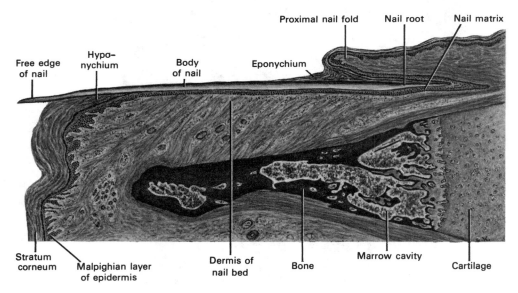

Figure 11.5. Drawing of a longitudinal section of a fingernail. (From Kelly DE, Wood RL, Enders AC: *Bailey's Textbook of Microscopic Anatomy*, ed 18. Baltimore, Williams & Wilkins, 1984.)

REVIEW TESTS
INTEGUMENT

DIRECTIONS: *One* or *more* of the given statements or completions is/are correct. Choose answer:

    A. if only **1**, **2**, and **3** are correct
    B. if only **1** and **3** are correct
    C. if only **2** and **4** are correct
    D. if only **4** is correct
    E. if **all** are correct

11.1. Intercellular bridges in the epidermis
1. are most common in the stratum granulosum
2. are most common in the stratum spinosum
3. represent sites where gap junctions are present between keratinocytes
4. represent sites where maculae adherentes are present between keratinocytes

11.2. Eccrine sweat glands
1. are not present in thick skin
2. release their secretion by the mechanism of holocrine secretion
3. have a narrow duct lined in part by myoepithelial cells
4. have a secretory portion that contains myoepithelial cells

11.3. A hair follicle
1. is always associated with a sweat gland
2. would not be present in thick skin
3. does not contain epithelial cells
4. is attached to the arrector pili muscle

11.4. Melanocytes
1. are pigment-producing cells in the skin
2. are located in the epidermis
3. transfer melanosomes to keratinocytes
4. give rise to keratinocytes

11.5. The stratum granulosum
1. contains melanosomes
2. lies superficial to the stratum lucidum
3. is the thickest layer of the epidermis in thick skin
4. contains keratohyalin granules

11.6. Sebaceous glands
1. are associated with hair follicles
2. employ the mechanism of merocrine secretion
3. produce a secretion called sebum
4. are present in thick skin

DIRECTIONS: The following questions or statements refer to the photomicrograph (Fig. 11.6). Select the *one* lettered structure in the labeled photomicrograph that *best* corresponds to the numbered phrase or description listed below. Each letter may be selected once, more than once, or not at all.

Figure 11.6. From Gartner LP, Hiatt JL: *Atlas of Histology*. Baltimore, Williams & Wilkins 1987.

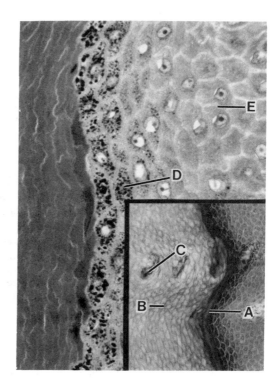

11.7. a layer seldom found in thin skin

11.8. stratum containing keratohyalin

11.9. the layer whose cells contain intercellular bridges

11.10. sweat gland duct in stratum corneum

DIRECTIONS: Each of the following statements contains five suggested completions. Choose the *one* that is *best* in each case.

11.11. Nails have each of the following features *except*:

A. an eponychium, or cuticle
B. a proximal, whitish, crescent-shaped lunula
C. a body (nail plate) that is composed of soft keratin
D. a nail matrix at their root that is responsible for nail growth
E. a hyponichium, where the skin is attached at the undersurface of the free border

11.12. Skin has all of the following components *except*

A. an epidermis
B. a dermis
C. a hypodermis
D. a stratified squamous keratinized epithelium
E. melanocytes in the stratum basale

11.13. The Langerhans cell

A. is commonly found in the dermis
B. originates from the ectoderm
C. functions as a sensory receptor for cold
D. plays an immunological role in the skin
E. functions as a pressure receptor

11.14. Meissner's corpuscles are found in the

A. epidermis
B. reticular layer of the dermis
C. hypodermis
D. papillary layer of the dermis
E. epidermal ridges

11.15. Thin skin

A. does not contain sweat glands
B. lacks a stratum corneum
C. is less abundant than thick skin
D. would not contain an arrector pili muscle
E. contains hair follicles

ANSWERS AND EXPLANATIONS

INTEGUMENT

11.1. C (2 and 4)
"Intercellular bridges" were described in the epidermis by early histologists who observed them between cells in the stratum spinosum. With the advent of the electron microscope, it was discovered that these intercellular bridges represent sites where desmosomes (maculae adherentes) attached adjacent cell processes.

11.2. D (4)
Eccrine sweat glands are found both in thick and thin skin. They release their secretion via the merocrine mechanism, and their narrow duct is lined by a stratified cuboidal epithelium. The secretory unit of an eccrine sweat gland consists of glandular epithelial cells, surrounded by an incomplete layer of underlying myoepithelial cells.

11.3. C (2 and 4)
A hair follicle encloses the root of each hair and is lined by epithelium. It is located only in thin skin and is not associated with eccrine sweat glands. The arrector pili muscle attaches each hair follicle to the more superficial papillary layer of the dermis. This muscle is arranged at such an angle that when it contracts it causes the hair to stand erect (forming goose flesh).

11.4. A (1, 2, and 3)
Melanocytes produce melanin pigment and transfer it to the keratinocytes. Early in development melanocytes migrate into the epidermis and form part of the basal cell layer. They do not give rise to keratinocytes.

11.5. D (4)
The stratum granulosum contains a number of dense keratohyalin granules. It lies just deep to the stratum lucidum and is a relatively thin layer of the epidermis in thick skin. It does not contain melanosomes, since they were destroyed by lysosomal enzymes in the stratum spinosum.

11.6. B (1 and 3)
Sebaceous glands have excretory ducts that open into the necks of hair follicles. They use the mechanism of holocrine secretion, which involves a breakdown of the secretory cells themselves, which are released along with their product. The cellular debris, along with the secretion itself, constitute the oily material known as sebum.

For questions **11.7** through **11.10**, refer to Figure 11.6.

11.7. A

11.8. D

11.9. E

11.10. C

11.11. C
The body of a nail is composed of hard, not soft, keratin. All of the other statements about nails are true.

11.12. C
The hypodermis is adipose connective tissue (superficial fascia) lying deep to the reticular layer of the dermis. It is not considered to be part of skin.

11.13. D

Langerhans cells in the epidermis function as antigen-presenting cells. They trap antigens that have penetrated the epidermis and transport them to regional lymph nodes where they are transferred to lymphocytes. In this way they provide an immune defense mechanism for the body.

11.14. D

Meissner's corpuscles are encapsulated nerve endings found in dermal papillae, which are part of the papillary layer of the dermis. Meissner's corpuscles function as receptors for fine touch.

11.15. E

In contrast to thick skin, which lacks hair follicles, thin skin contains many of them. All of the other statements about thin skin are false.

12
Respiratory System

Function of Respiratory System

—is to provide oxygen to the tissues of the body in exchange for carbon dioxide.
—is accomplished through two major divisions of the system:

  —conducting portion: airways that deliver air to the lungs.
  —respiratory portion: structures within the lung where gaseous exchange occurs.

Conducting Portion of Respiratory System

—delivers air to the respiratory tissue.
—conducting airways include the nose, pharynx, larynx, trachea, bonchi, and bronchioles, down to and including the terminal bronchioles.
—these parts of the system warm, moisten, and filter the air before it reaches the respiratory tissue.

Respiratory Portion of Respiratory System

—is where exchange of gases takes place.
—includes the respiratory bronchioles, alveolar ducts, alveolar sacs, and alveoli.
—these parts of the system are intrapulmonary and contain alveoli.

Nasal Cavity

Nares

—nostrils, whose outermost portions are lined by extensions of skin.
—this keratinized epithelium is stratified squamous and contains sweat glands, hair follicles, and sebaceous glands.

Vestibule

—is the first portion of the nasal cavity.
—contains vibrissae (thick short hairs) that filter out large particles from the inspired air.
—posteriorly, the lining changes to respiratory epithelium (pseudostratified ciliated columnar epithelium with goblet cells).
—lamina propria is vascular (contains many venous plexuses) and has a number of seromucous glands.

Olfactory Epithelium

Location

—roof of nasal cavity, on either side of the nasal septum and onto the superior nasal conchae.

—consists of a tall pseudostratified columnar epithelium with three cell types: olfactory, supporting, and basal cells.

Olfactory Cells

—are bipolar nerve cells characterized by a bulbous projection (olfactory vesicle) from which several modified cilia extend.
—olfactory cilia, which act as receptors, are nonmotile and very long. Their proximal one-third contains a typical axoneme but their distal two-thirds is composed of nine peripheral singlets surrounding two central singlets.

Supporting (sustentacular) Cells

—possess nuclei that are more apically located than those in the other two cell types.
—have many microvilli and a prominent terminal web.

Basal Cells

—rest on the basal lamina but do not extend to the surface.
—form an imcomplete layer of cells.
—are believed to be regenerative for all three cell types.

Lamina Propria

—contains many veins, unmyelinated nerves, and Bowman's glands.

Bowman's Glands

—produce a watery serous secretion that is released onto the olfactory epithelial surface via narrow ducts.
—olfactory stimuli dissolve in this material and are carried away by the secretion to prepare the receptors for new stimuli.

Pharynx

Characteristics

—divided into nasal, oral, and laryngeal portions.
—nasopharynx is lined by respiratory epithelium.
—oropharynx and laryngopharynx are lined by stratified squamous nonkeratinized epithelium.
—connective tissue beneath the epithelium contains mucous and serous glands as well as an abundance of lymphoid tissue.

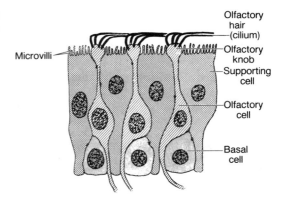

Figure 12.1. Diagram of the olfactory epithelium. (From Karuse WJ, Cutts JH: *Concise Text of Histology*, ed 2. Baltimore, Williams & Wilkins, 1986.)

Olfactory hair (cilium)
Olfactory knob
Supporting cell
Olfactory cell
Basal cell
Microvilli

Larynx
Characteristics
—connects the pharynx with the trachea.
—wall is supported by hyaline cartilages (thyroid, cricoid, lower part of arytenoids) and elastic cartilages (epiglottis, corniculate, and tips of arytenoids).
—remainder of wall contains striated muscle and connective tissue with glands.

Vocal Cords
—consist of skeletal muscle (the vocalis), the vocal ligament (formed by a band of elastic fibers), and a covering of stratified squamous nonkeratinized epithelium.
—muscles within the larynx contract and change the size of the opening between the vocal cords, which affects the pitch of the sounds caused by air passing through the larynx.

Lining Epithelium
—changes to respiratory epithelium at base of epiglottis, inferior to the vocal cords.
—respiratory epithelium lines air passages down through trachea and primary bronchi.

Vestibular Fold
—lies superior to the vocal cord.
—is a fold of loose connective tissue containing glands and lymphoid aggregations.
—is covered by respiratory epithelium.

Trachea and Extrapulmonary Bronchi
Hyaline Cartilage
—supports walls of trachea and extrapulmonary bronchi.
—cartilages are C shaped, with their open ends facing posteriorly.
—smooth muscle (trachealis) extends between open ends of the cartilage.
—dense fibroelastic connective tissue is present, superior and inferior to each cartilage, which facilitates the elongation of the trachea during inhalation.

Respiratory Epithelium
—lines the lumen of the trachea and extrapulmonary bronchi.
—in the human it consists of the following cell types:

Ciliated Cells
—have long actively motile extensions that beat in the direction of the pharynx.
—thus delicate lung tissue is protected from possible damage by inhaled particulate matter.
—ciliated cells also contain microvilli.

Mucous Cells
—are of two varieties: mature goblet cells and small mucous granule cells.

Mature Goblet Cell
—is best known because of its shape.
—is filled with large mucous droplets that are secreted to trap inhaled particles.

Small Mucous Granule Cell
—sometimes called "brush" cell because of its many microvilli.
—contains varying numbers of small mucous granules.

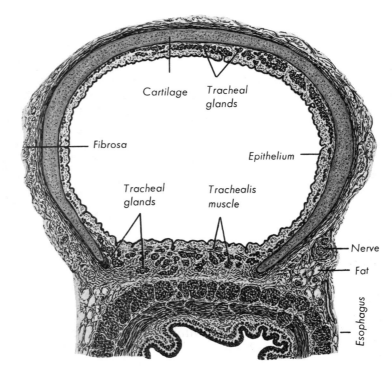

Figure 12.2. Drawing of a cross section of the trachea and part of the esophagus. (From Kelly DE, Wood RL, Enders AC: *Bailey's Textbook of Microscopic Anatomy*, ed 18. Baltimore, Williams & Wilkins, 1984.)

—actively divides and thus might be able to replace recently desquamated cells; might also be a goblet cell that has secreted its mucus.

Enteroendocrine Cells

—(APUD cells, small granule cells) also form part of the epithelium.
—contain many small granules concentrated in their basal cytoplasm.
—various types of enteroendocrine cells synthesize different polypeptide hormones.
—these cells exert a local affect on nearby structures and cell types (paracrine regulation).

Short (basal) Cells

—rest on the basal lamina but do not extend to the lumen, making epithelium pseudo-stratified.
—are able to divide.

Basement Membrane

—is a very thick layer that underlies the epithelium.

Lamina Propria

—a thin layer of connective tissue that lies beneath the basement membrane.
—elastic fibers run longitudinally and separate the lamina propria from the sub-mucosa.

Submucosa

—contains many seromucous glands.

Adventitia

—forms the outer layer of the trachea.

—contains C-shaped cartilages.

Intrapulmonary Bronchi (Secondary Bronchi)

Origin

—arise from subdivisions of the primary bronchi and divide many times.

—have irregular cartilage plates in their walls.

—respiratory epithelium lines the lumina of the intrapulmonary bronchi.

Lamina Propria

—is separated from the submucosa by layers of spiraling smooth muscle.

Glands (seromucous)

—are present in the submucosa.

Bronchioles

General Characteristics

—bronchioles measure 1 mm or less in diameter and have no cartilage in their walls.

—smooth muscle replaces the cartilage plates, and glands are not present.

—its lining epithelium varies from ciliated columnar with goblet cells (in the primary bronchioles) to ciliated cuboidal with secretory (Clara) cells (in terminal and respiratory bronchioles).

Terminal Bronchiole

—is the most distal part of the conducting portion of the respiratory system.

—is lined by a simple cuboidal epithelium consisting of Clara (secretory) cells and ciliated cells.

—Clara cells also contain an abundance of smooth endoplasmic reticulum (whose enzymes may be involved in metabolizing toxins from the inspired air).

Respiratory Bronchiole

—marks the transition between the conducting and respiratory portion of the system.

—its wall is interrupted by alveoli, which makes it the first portion of the pulmonary tree in which gaseous exchange takes place.

—its remaining wall is lined by a simple cuboidal epithelium consisting of Clara cells and ciliated cells.

Alveolar Duct

Characteristics

—linear passageway continuous with the respiratory bronchiole.

—its wall consists of closely spaced alveoli that are separated from one another only by an interalveolar septum.

—smooth muscle is present in the septum at the opening of adjacent alveoli.

—alveolar duct is most distal portion of the respiratory system to contain smooth muscle in its wall.

—an attenuated simple squamous epithelium (consisting of type I and type II pneumocytes) lines the alveolar duct.

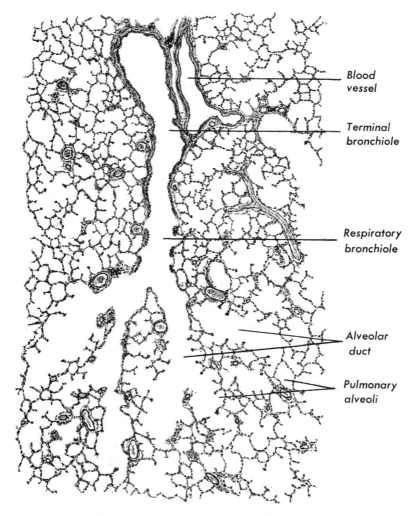

Figure 12.3. Drawing of a section of the lung. (From Kelly DE, Wood RL, Enders AC: *Bailey's Textbook of Microscopic Anatomy*, ed 18. Baltimore, Williams & Wilkins, 1984.)

Alveolar Sac

Characteristics

—an expanded irregular space at the distal end of an alveolar duct, whose wall consists of adjacent alveoli.

Alveoli

Characteristics

—permit gaseous exchange between air and blood (oxygen from air to blood, and carbon dioxide from blood to air).

—communicate with each other via alveolar pores (of Kohn).

—rims of the openings into alveoli contain elastic fibers and supportive reticular fibers.

—alveoli are lined by a highly attenuated simple squamous epithelium composed of two cell types.

Type I Pneumocyte

—(type I alveolar cell) covers about 95% of alveolar surface.
—forms part of the blood-gas barrier.
—has an extremely thin cytoplasm (can be less than 80 nm in thickness).
—forms tight junctions with neighboring cells.
—is not able to divide.

Type II Pneumocyte

—(type II alveolar cell, great alveolar cell, granular pneumocyte, septal cell) is low cuboidal and is located most often near septal intersections.
—bulging free surface contains short microvilli that are located peripherally.
—synthesizes pulmonary surfactant, which it stores in lamellar bodies in its cytoplasm.
—release of surfactant from the lamellar bodies produces a monomolecular film that spreads over the alveolar surface.
—is able to divide and regenerate both cell types in the alveolar epithelium.
—forms tight junctions with neighboring cells.

Alveolar Macrophage

—(dust cell, alveolar phagocyte) is the principal mononuclear phagocyte of the alveolar surface.
—removes inhaled dust, bacteria, and other particulate matter and is a vital line of defense in the lung.
—when filled with debris it migrates to the bronchioles and is carried via ciliary action to the upper airways and pharynx, where it is swallowed.
—another exit route is to migrate into the interstitium and leave via lymphatics.

Interalveolar Septum

Characteristics

—septum is the wall, or partition, between two alveoli.
—continuous capillaries occupy its central (interior) region, and an attenuated simple squamous epithelium lines the alveoli bordering its outer surfaces.
—elastin and reticular fibers are present in some of the thicker regions of the septal wall.
—elsewhere the septum constitutes the site of the blood-gas barrier.

Blood-Gas Barrier

—is the barrier to diffusion of gases between the alveolar air and the blood.
—in thinnest areas it consists of the following components:

1. layer of surfactant
2. thin epithelium of the type I pneumocyte
3. fused basal laminae of the type I pneumocyte and capillary endothelium
4. endothelium of the continuous capillary

—average distance across the barrier is about 0.5 μm.
—in areas where the two basal laminae fuse, to eliminate the thin interstitial space, the distance across the barrier is reduced to 0.2 μm or less.

Vascular Supply of Lungs

Pulmonary Artery

—carries blood to the lungs to be oxygenated.
—enters the root of each lung and extends branches along the divisions of the bronchial tree.

Pulmonary Veins

—run independently of the arteries in the intersegmental connective tissue.
—after leaving the lobules of the lung the veins come into close association with branches of the bronchial tree.
—from this point to the root of the lung the veins accompany the bronchi.
—thus branches of the pulmonary artery and vein follow branches of the bronchial tree, except within the lobules, where only arteries follow the bronchioles.

Lung Lobules

Characteristics

—each bronchiole that arises from a bronchus enters what is known as a lung lobule.
—lobules are shaped somewhat like a pyramid, having an apex and a base, but they vary greatly in size and shape.
—an incomplete septum separates each lobule from its neighbor.
—lymphatics run within the dense connective tissue but are not present within the interalveolar wall.

Nerve Supply

Nerve Fibers

—from both divisions of the autonomic nervous system innervate the smooth muscle of bronchi and bronchioles.
—axons have been demonstrated in thicker parts of the interalveolar septa.

Breathing

Characteristics

—during inspiration the thoracic cage enlarges, becoming deeper, wider, and longer.
—large amounts of elastic tissue within the lungs permit extensive expansion and relaxation to occur.
—each lung is enclosed in a pleural sac and the pleural space is under negative pressure.
—as the thoracic wall increases in size, the visceral pleura, which is firmly attached to the lungs, is also drawn outward.
—this decreases the air pressure within the lungs and air is drawn into them.
—since air has been inspired, the elastic tissue in the lungs is stretched.
—the elastic recoil is enough to expel air from the lungs, decreasing the thoracic cage to its initial size.

REVIEW TESTS

RESPIRATORY SYSTEM

DIRECTIONS: *One* or *more* of the given statements or completions is/are correct. Choose answer:

   A. if only **1**, **2**, and **3** are correct
   B. if only **1** and **3** are correct
   C. if only **2** and **4** are correct
   D. if only **4** is correct
   E. if **all** are correct

12.1. The olfactory epithelium
1. is located at the base of the nasal cavity
2. contains bipolar nerve cells
3. contains Bowman's glands
4. has modified cilia that act as receptors

12.2. Terminal bronchioles
1. are part of the conducting portion of the respiratory system
2. function in gaseous exchange
3. contain ciliated cells
4. have cartilage plates present in their walls

12.3. The larynx
1. is part of the pharynx
2. contains vestibular folds
3. contains fibrocartilage
4. contains vocal cords

12.4. The trachea
1. contains irregular cartilage plates in its wall
2. contains skeletal muscle in its wall
3. is lined by an epithelium containing only two cell types
4. has a thick basement membrane underlying its epithelium

12.5. Bronchi
1. contain seromucous glands in their submucosa
2. contain cartilage in their walls
3. are lined by an epithelium containing ciliated cells
4. have secretory (Clara) cells as part of their epithelium

12.6. Alveoli
1. contain elastic fibers in their walls
2. permit gaseous exchange between the air and the blood
3. contain reticular fibers in their walls
4. are lined by a simple squamous epithelium

12.7. The respiratory bronchiole
1. permits limited gaseous exchange
2. does not have alveoli forming part of its wall
3. contains Clara cells in its lining epithelium
4. forms part of the conducting portion of the respiratory system

DIRECTIONS: The following questions or statements refer to the electron micrograph (Fig. 12.4). Select the *one* lettered structure that is most closely associated with each of the following descriptive phrases or items. Each letter may be used once, more than once, or not at all.

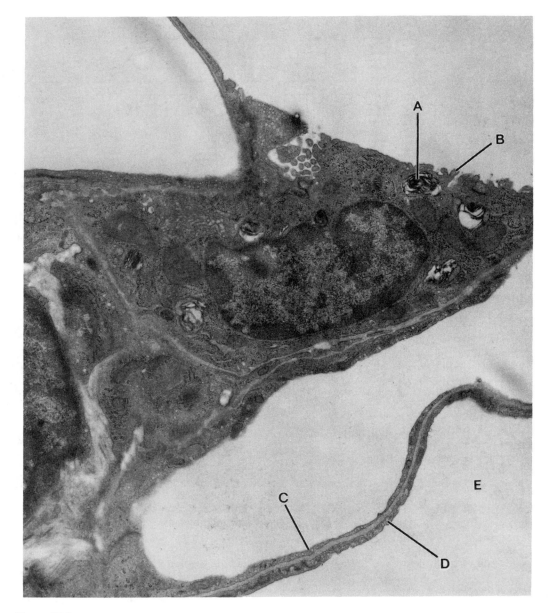

Figure 12.4.

12.8. microvillus

12.9. process of a type I pneumocyte

12.10. contains surfactant

12.11. alveolus

12.12. endothelium lining a capillary

DIRECTIONS: Each of the following questions contains five suggested answers. Choose the *one* that is *best* in each case.

12.13. Olfactory hairs are
A. actively motile cilia
B. appendages of sustentacular cells
C. part of specialized bipolar nerve cells
D. found in respiratory epithelium lining the nares
E. present in Bowman's glands

12.14. Alveoli are present in all of the following locations *except*
A. in alveolar sacs
B. in respiratory bronchioles
C. in alveolar ducts
D. in terminal bronchioles
E. where the blood-air barrier exists

12.15. Intrapulmonary bronchi
A. have C-shaped cartilages in their walls
B. lack smooth muscle
C. are lined in part by Clara cells
D. have irregular cartilage plates in their walls
E. are lined by a simple squamous epithelium

12.16. Alveolar macrophages
A. are multinucleated
B. are phagocytic
C. originate from blood neutrophils
D. are not present in the interalveolar septum
E. are identical to type II pneumocytes

ANSWERS AND EXPLANATIONS

RESPIRATORY SYSTEM

12.1. C (2 and 4)
The olfactory epithelium is located in the roof of the nasal cavity. It contains bipolar nerve cells with modified nonmotile cilia that serve as receptors for smell. Bowman's glands, which lie in the lamina propria beneath this epithelium, produce a watery fluid that moistens the olfactory surface.

12.2. B (1 and 3)
Terminal bronchioles mark the end of the conducting portion of the respiratory system. They are lined by an epithelium composed of two cell types: secretory (Clara) cells and ciliated cells. They lack alveoli and contain no cartilage.

12.3. C (2 and 4)
The vocal cords are important structural parts of the larynx. They are lined by stratified squamous nonkeratinized epithelium. In the connective tissue deep to the epithelium is skeletal muscle (the vocalis). The vestibular folds lie superior to the vocal cords and are separated from them by an indentation, or recess. The vestibular folds consist of loose connective tissue lined by a respiratory epithelium. Hyaline and elastic cartilages form part of the larynx.

12.4. D (4)
The pseudostratified ciliated columnar epithelium rests upon a thick basement membrane. The trachea contains C-shaped cartilages with smooth muscle present between their ends.

12.5. A (1, 2, and 3)
Bronchi have submucosal glands and contain hyaline cartilage. They are lined by respiratory epithelium, which contains ciliated cells. Clara cells are not present in bronchi, since they are found only in the bronchioles.

12.6. E (all are correct)
The walls of alveoli are composed primarily of reticular and elastic fibers. The function of the alveoli is to permit gaseous exchange, and their thin epithelium is classified as simple squamous.

12.7. B (1 and 3)
Respiratory bronchioles have alveoli interrupting their walls, so some gaseous exchange takes place at this level. The remainder of their wall is lined by a simple cuboidal epithelium consisting of Clara cells and ciliated cells.

For questions **12.8** through **12.12**, refer to the labeled electron micrograph (Fig. 12.4).

12.8. B

12.9. D

12.10. A

12.11. E

12.12. C

12.13. C
Olfactory hairs are part of the specialized bipolar receptor nerve cells in the olfactory epithelium. They are long, nonmotile, modified cilia that are found exclusively in this epithelium.

12.14. D
Alveoli are not present in the terminal bronchioles, which constitute the last component of the conducting portion of the respiratory system.

184

12.15. D

Irregular cartilage plates are characteristic of the intrapulmonary bronchi. The C-shaped cartilages end with the primary bronchi. All bronchi contain smooth muscle and are lined by respiratory epithelium or a simple columnar ciliated epithelium.

12.16. B

Alveolar macrophages are scavengers of the alveolar surface and are avidly phagocytic. They originate from blood monocytes. They are unrelated to type II pneumocytes and are not present in the interalveolar septum.

13

Digestive System I: Oral Cavity

Digestive System

—begins at the oral cavity.

Oral Cavity

—is the site where food is moistened, chewed, and compacted into small fragments, known as boluses, which are propelled into the pharynx to be swallowed.

Oral Region

—includes the lips, teeth (and associated structures), palate, tongue, tonsils, as well as the major salivary glands (to be discussed in Chapter 15).

Pharynx

—is continuous with the oral cavity at its proximal end and with the esophagus and larynx at its distal end.

Lips

Surfaces

External Surface

—covered with thin skin having hair follicles, sebaceous glands, and sweat glands.

Vermillion Zone

—the red portion of the lip, is covered by stratified squamous keratinized epithelium having deep epidermal ridges that interdigitate with high dermal papillae.

—hair follicles and glands are not associated with this region, although sebaceous glands may occasionally be present.

Internal Surface

—lined by stratified squamous nonkeratinized epithelium. The mucosa and submucosa contain minor seromucous salivary glands.

Core

—consists of dense irregular collagenous connective tissue enveloping skeletal muscle (chiefly the orbicularis oris).

Teeth and Associated Structures

Teeth

Dentition

—deciduous dentition (milk teeth) consists of 20 teeth that are exfoliated between 6 and 13 years of age.

—succedaneous (permanent) dentition, composed of 32 teeth, replaces the deciduous teeth by the 18th to 20th year of life.

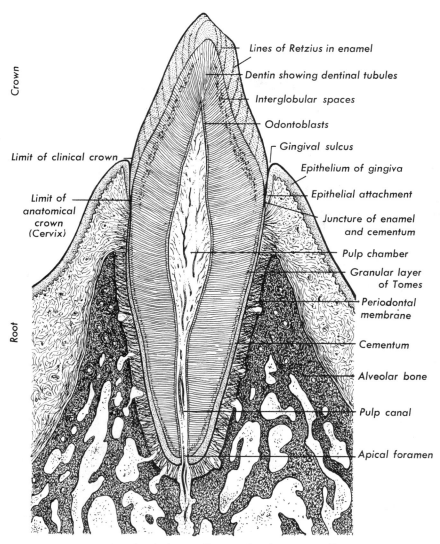

Figure 13.1. Diagram of a section of an incisor and its associated structures. (From Kelly DE, Wood RL, Enders AC: *Bailey's Textbook of Microscopic Anatomy*, ed 18. Baltimore, Williams & Wilkins, 1984.)

Anatomy

—each tooth is divided into an enamel-covered crown, a cementum-covered root, and a cervix, where the cementum and enamel meet.
—bulk of the tooth is composed of dentin, surrounding the central pulp chamber, and root canal (housing the pulp).

Early Tooth Development

—begins with the formation of the epithelially derived, horseshoe-shaped dental laminae between the sixth and seventh week of development.
—epithelial-mesenchymal interaction is responsible for the formation of 10 enamel organs at discrete points along the lingual aspect of each dental lamina.

Enamel Organs

—mature through the bud, cap, and the bell stages of odontogenesis.

Cap Stage

—mitotic activity of the bud increases its size, forming a cap-shaped enamel organ.
—composed of three layers: the convex outer enamel epithelium (OEE), the concave inner enamel epithelium (IEE), and the intervening stellate reticulum (SR).
—OEE and IEE meet at the cervical loop, establishing the distal aspect of the concavity filled by closely packed ectomesenchymal cells (derived from neural crest), collectively referred to as the *dental papilla*.
—additional ectomesenchymal cells surround the tooth germ and form a membrane known as the *dental sac* (follicle).
—succedaneous lamina, derived from the dental lamina, is also initiated at this time.

Bell Stage

—mitotic activity enlarges the cap and concomitantly forms a new layer of cells, the stratum intermedium (SI), located between the SR and the IEE.
—is composed of four layers and possesses a deep concavity filled with dental papilla.
—cells of the IEE elongate and differentiate, becoming tall columnar preameloblasts.
—cells at the periphery of the dental papilla respond by elongating and differentiating into tall columnar preodontoblasts.

Apposition

—the preodontoblasts and preameloblasts become functional to elaborate dentin and enamel matrix, respectively.

Root Formation

—after completion of the crown, the cervical loop elongates distally, forming an epithelial collar, Hertwig's epithelial root sheath (HERS).

Epithelial Diaphragm

—the medial extension of HERS, functions in delimiting the site of radicular (root) dentin formation.
—also determines the size, shape, and number of roots the tooth will possess.

HERS

—disintegrates during the formation of the root, and ectomesenchymal cells from the dental sac migrate through the newly created spaces.
—ectomesenchymal cells reach the radicular dentin, differentiate into cementoblasts, and elaborate cementum matrix.

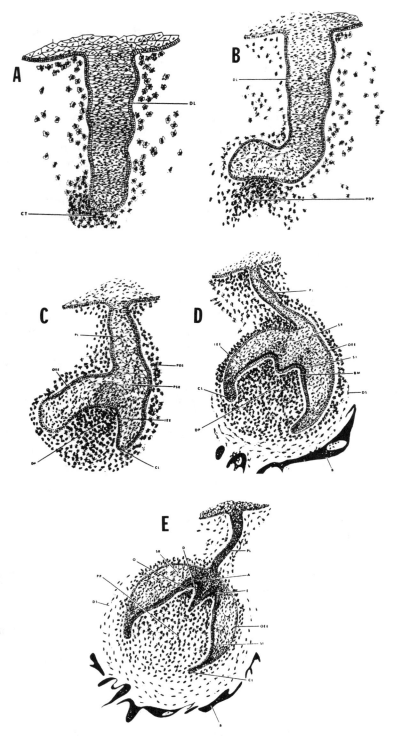

Figure 13.2. Diagrams of the various stages of tooth development. **A**, dental lamina stage. **B**, bud stage. **C**, cap stage. **D**, bell stage. **E**, appositional stage. [From Hiatt JL, Gartner LP, Provenza DV: Molar development in the Mongolian gerbil (*Meriones unguiculatus*). *Am J Anat* 141:1–22, 1974.]

Tissues of the Tooth

Enamel

—is the hardest substance of the body. It is composed of 96% mineralized material (calcium hydroxyapatite) and 4% bound water and enamel protein, a substance related to keratin.

—formative cells are not associated with enamel subsequent to eruption.

Dentin

—is similar in organic composition to bone.

—is composed of 65 to 70% calcium hydroxyapatite, and its organic matrix is mostly collagen, proteoglycans, and glycoproteins.

Odontoblast Processes

—are located within tunnel-like dentinal tubules throughout the dentin.

Dentinal Tubules

—describe S-shaped curves extending from the dentinoenamel (or dentinocemental) junction to the pulp.

Cementum

—is composed of 45 to 50% calcium hydroxyapatite, with an organic component consisting of collagen, glycoproteins, and proteoglycans.

Cells

—known as cementoblasts and cementocytes are associated with cementum. Cementum housing cementocytes in lacunae is referred to as *cellular cementum*, whereas cementum without cementocytes is known as *acellular cementum*.

Pulp

—is located in the pulp chamber.

—is a gelatinous, embryonic-like connective tissue, equipped with a rich vascular, neural, and lymphatic supply.

—has four zones: the most peripheral odontoblastic zone, a cell-free zone, a cell-rich zone, and the pulp core.

Periodontal Ligament

Fibers

—are almost exclusively collagen, although according to some, preelastic (oxytalan) fibers may also be present.

Principal Fiber Bundles

—are composed of thick collagen bundles that suspend the tooth in its alveolus.

—extend from cementum to bone (and their terminals are embedded as Sharpey's fibers in both).

—five principal fiber groups are the alveolar crest, horizontal, oblique, apical, and interradicular.

Cells

—are cementoblasts, fibroblasts, mast cells, extravasated white blood cells, occasional fat cells, osteoblasts, and cell rests of Malassez (HERS epithelial remnants).

Nerve and Vascular Supply

—is present in abundance.

Gingiva

Epithelium
—stratified squamous keratinized (parakeratinized = partially keratinized) with long rete ridges (pegs).

Connective Tissue
—is dense irregular collagenous, with high connective tissue papillae.
—collagen is arranged in principal fiber bundles, known as dentogingival, dentoperiosteal, alveologingival, circular, and transseptal.

Alveolar Bone

Structure
—consists of an inner and an outer layer of compact bone with an intervening cancellous bone, the spongiosa.

Cribriform Plate (lamina dura)
—is the inner layer that surrounds the root of the tooth.
—fibers of the periodontal ligament are embedded in this region, via Sharpey's fibers, thus suspending the tooth in its bony alveolus.
—blood vessels arising from the spongiosa enter the periodontal ligament via perforations in the cribriform plate.

Cortical plate
—is the thick outer layer.

Palate

Hard Palate
—nasal aspect is covered by pseudostratified ciliated columnar epithelium.
—oral aspect is lined by stratified squamous keratinized (parakeratinized) epithelium whose long rete ridges interdigitate with tall connective tissue papillae of the lamina propria.

Periosteum
—of the bony shelf is firmly bound to the collagen fiber bundles of the palatal mucosa.
—mucosa contains adipose tissue anterolaterally and mucous minor salivary glands posterolaterally.

Soft Palate
—nasal aspect is covered by pseudostratified ciliated columnar epithelium.
—oral aspect is lined by stratified squamous (nonkeratinized) epithelium.

Core
—is composed of thick bundles of skeletal muscle fibers and contains mucous minor salivary glands.

Tongue

Divisions
—the tongue is subdivided into an anterior two-thirds and a posterior one-third.

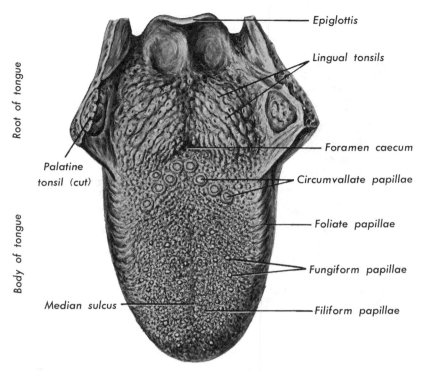

Figure 13.3. Drawing of the dorsal surface of a human tongue. (From Kelly DE, Wood RL, Enders AC: *Bailey's Textbook of Microscopic Anatomy*, ed 18. Baltimore, Williams & Wilkins, 1984.)

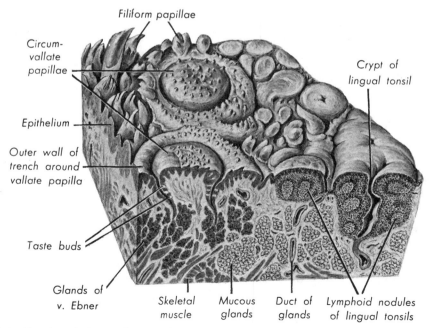

Figure 13.4. Drawing of circumvallate papillae and lingual tonsils. (From Kelly DE, Wood RL, Enders AC: *Bailey's Textbook of Microscopic Anatomy*, ed 18. Baltimore, Williams & Wilkins, 1984.)

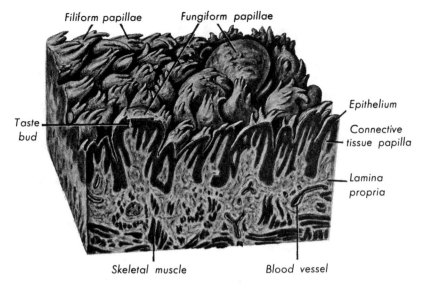

Figure 13.5. Drawing of fungiform and filiform papillae. (From Kelly DE, Wood RL, Enders, AC: *Bailey's Textbook of Microscopic Anatomy*, ed 18. Baltimore, Williams & Wilkins, 1984.)

Sulcus Terminalis
—a V-shaped depression whose posteriorly pointing apex ends in a shallow pit, the foramen cecum, which separates the two regions from one another.

Anterior Two-Thirds

Dorsal Surface
—is covered by stratified squamous keratinized (parakeratinized) epithelium.
—presents four types of lingual papillae: filiform, fungiform, foliate, and circumvallate.

Filiform Papillae
—are short, narrow, pointed structures that project above the surface of the tongue.
—cornified surface permits the tongue to scrape material off a surface.
—connective tissue cores, as in all lingual papillae, form secondary papillae as they interdigitate with the rete ridges of the overlying epithelium.

Fungiform Papillae
—are mushroom-shaped structures that project above the surface of the tongue.
—epithelium on the dorsal surface of these papillae contain occasional taste buds.

Foliate Papillae
—are located on the lateral aspect of the tongue.
—are not well developed in human adults, although they may be functional in neonates, where taste buds have been noted.
—appear as shallow, longitudinal furrows into which the serous glands of von Ebner drain.

Circumvallate Papillae
—are 10 to 15 in number.
—are located in front of the sulcus terminalis, embedded into the surface of the tongue.

—are surrounded by a moat-like furrow. The lateral surface of the papilla contains taste buds in its epithelium.

—glands of von Ebner deliver their serous secretions into the base of the furrow, thus assisting in the process of taste.

Taste Buds

—are small, intraepithelial structures that function in the perception of the four taste sensations: salt, sour, bitter, and sweet.

—are composed of three different types of cells in humans: sustentacular, neuroepithelial, and basal cells.

—electron micrographs do not demonstrate a functional difference between sustentacular and neuroepithelial cells, which have been named type I and type II cells.

—electron micrographs display long microvilli in both cell types (the taste hairs described by light microscopists), which pass through the taste pore to be bathed in saliva.

—basal cells are believed to be regenerative.

Muscular Core

—constitutes the bulk of the tongue.

—is composed of several bundles of skeletal muscle fibers that cross each other in three perpendicular planes.

—epimysia of these muscle bundles are interlaced with the connective tissue elements of the lamina propria and/or submucosa.

Minor Salivary Glands

—are interspersed among the muscle fibers, the serous glands of von Ebner, the mixed anterior glands of Blandin-Nuhn, and the mucous posterior lingual glands.

Ventral Surface

—is lined by stratified (nonkeratinized) squamous epithelium.

—lamina propria and submucosa are both composed of dense irregular collagenous connective tissue.

Posterior One-Third

—lingual tonsil lies in the posterior one-third of the tongue.

Tonsils

Palatine Tonsils

—are lymphatic aggregates located between the palatopharyngeal and palatoglossal arches.

—crypts, which frequently contain debris, are formed from deep invaginations of the stratified squamous epithelium covering of the tonsils.

—lymphatic nodules exhibit germinal centers (secondary nodules).

—connective tissue capsule surrounds the deep aspect of the palatine tonsil.

Pharyngeal Tonsil

—is located in the posterior wall of the nasopharynx.

—is covered by a pseudostratified ciliated columnar epithelium that contains several folds.

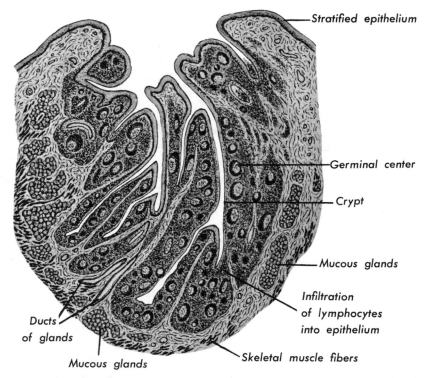

Figure 13.6. Drawing of a section of palatine tonsils. (From Kelly DE, Wood RL, Enders AC: *Bailey's Textbook of Microscopic Anatomy*, ed 18. Baltimore, Williams & Wilkins, 1984.)

—glands located in the connective tissue deep to the tonsilar capsule, deliver their seromucous secretions into the folds.

Lingual Tonsils
—are covered by a stratified squamous epithelium, which forms deep crypts, frequently containing cellular debris.
—ducts of mucous glands often open into the base of these crypts.

REVIEW TESTS
DIGESTIVE SYSTEM I

DIRECTIONS: *One* or *more* of the given statements or completions is/are correct. Choose answer:

A. if only **1**, **2**, and **3** are correct
B. if only **1** and **3** are correct
C. if only **2** and **4** are correct
D. if only **4** is correct
E. if **all** are correct

13.1. The type of epithelium associated with the lip is/are
1. stratified squamous nonkeratinized
2. pseudostratified ciliated columnar
3. stratified squamous keratinized
4. stratified cuboidal

13.2. The bell stage of tooth development is characterized by
1. stratum intermedium
2. stratum granulosum
3. stellate reticulum
4. Hertwig's epithelial root sheath

13.3. The appositional stage of tooth development is characterized by the presence of
1. an epithelial diaphragm
2. an alveolus
3. the dental sac
4. enamel

13.4. The cribriform plate belongs to the
1. gingiva
2. periodontal ligament
3. pulp
4. alveolus

13.5. Which of the following papillae have taste buds?
1. circumvallate
2. fungiform
3. foliate
4. filiform

DIRECTIONS: The following questions or statements refer to the photomicrographs (Figs. 13.7 and 13.8) below. The letters on the figures are answers to the numbered items appearing below each photomicrograph. For each numbered item select the *one* letter that *best* corresponds to that item. Each letter may be used once, more than once, or not at all.

Figure 13.7. From Gartner LP, Hiatt JL: *Atlas of Histology.* Baltimore, Williams & Wilkins, 1987.

13.6. stratified squamous nonkeratinized epithelium

13.7. taste bud

13.8. glands of von Ebner

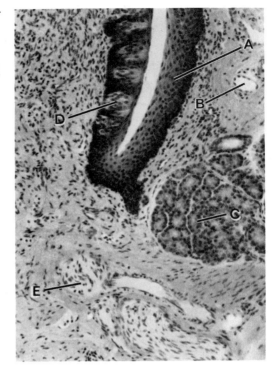

Figure 13.8. From Gartner LP, Hiatt JL: *Atlas of Histology.* Baltimore, Williams & Wilkins, 1987.

13.9. enamel

13.10. dentin

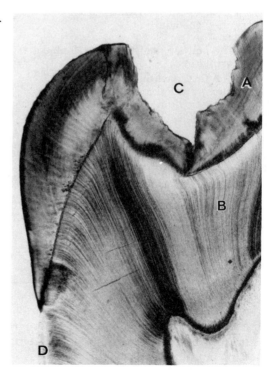

DIRECTIONS: Each of the following statements contains five suggested completions. Choose the *one* that is *best* in each case.

13.11. Odontoblastic processes are located in
A. cementum
B. enamel
C. dentin
D. the crown only
E. the root only

13.12. One of the following statements is *not* true:
A. Cementum may possess lacunae.
B. The organic fibers of enamel are collagenous in nature.
C. The organic fibers of dentin are collagenous in nature.
D. Calcium hydroxyapatite constitutes 45 to 50% of cementum.
E. The enamel of an erupted tooth is not associated with regenerative cells.

13.13. One of the following is not a zone of the pulp:
A. vermillion zone
B. odontoblastic zone
C. cell-free zone
D. cell-rich zone
E. core

13.14. The principal fiber bundles of the periodontal ligament
A. are composed of elastin
B. extend from cementum to enamel
C. extend from dentin to cementum
D. are composed of collagen
E. extend from one tooth to the next

13.15. The cribriform plate
A. is the inner layer of the alveolar bone
B. is the outer layer of the alveolar bone
C. does not possess Sharpey's fibers
D. is also known as the spongiosa
E. is composed of cancellous bone

13.16. One of the following is *not* true concerning the pharyngeal tonsil:
A. It is composed mostly of lymphoid aggregates.
B. It is covered by stratified squamous epithelium.
C. The epithelium is invaginated to form folds.
D. It does not possess tonsillar crypts.
E. It possesses a capsule.

ANSWERS AND EXPLANATIONS

DIGESTIVE SYSTEM I

13.1. B (1 and 3)
The lip is covered by skin on its external aspect and lined by a moist mucosa on its internal aspect. Epidermis is stratified squamous keratinized epithelium, whereas the moist mucosa of the internal aspect of the lip is stratified squamous nonkeratinized.

13.2. B (1 and 3)
The bell stage of tooth development is composed of four layers: outer enamel epithelium, inner enamel epithelium, stellate reticulum, and stratum intermedium. Hertwig's epithelial root sheath appears during root formation. The stratum granulosum is one of the layers of the epidermis and has nothing to do with tooth development.

13.3. D (4)
The term *apposition* refers to the elaboration of dentin by odontoblasts and enamel by ameloblasts. The epithelial diaphragm appears during the formation of the root of the tooth. The alveolus and dental sac begin to be formed during the cap stage of odontogenesis.

13.4. D (4)
The term *cribriform plate* refers to that portion of the alveolus that immediately surrounds the root of the tooth. Principal fiber groups of the periodontal ligament attach to the cribriform plate via Sharpey's fibers, but the cribriform plate is not considered a part of that structure. The gingiva and pulp have no connection to the cribriform plate.

13.5. A (1, 2, and 3)
Taste buds are found along the circumvallate and fungiform papillae at all stages in the human. Foliate papillae contain taste buds in the human neonate. Filiform papillae never contain taste buds.

For questions **13.6** to **13.8**, refer to a section of a circumvallate papilla (Fig. 13.7).

13.6. A, stratified squamous nonkeratinized epithelium

13.7. D, taste bud

13.8. C, glands of von Ebner

For questions **13.9** to **13.10**, refer to a ground section of a tooth (Fig. 13.8).

13.9. A, enamel

13.10. B, dentin

13.11. C
Coronal and radicular dentin both possess hollow, tunnel-like dentinal tubules that contain odontoblastic processes.

13.12. B
The question requires identification of the incorrect statement. Enamel does not possess collagen fibers; instead its organic fibers are known as enamel protein, a substance similar to keratin.

13.13. A
The question requires identification of the incorrect statement. The vermillion zone is not a region of the pulp. It is the red portion of the lip.

13.14. D
The principal fiber bundles of the periodontal ligament, composed of collagen fibers, suspend the tooth in its alveolus. Therefore these fiber bundles extend from the bony alveolus (cribriform plate) to the cementum on the root of the tooth. The fibers that extend from one tooth to the next are the transseptal fibers of the gingiva.

13.15. A
The cribriform plate, the inner layer of the alveolus, is composed of compact bone. The

principal fiber groups of the periodontal ligament attach to the cribriform plate via Sharpey's fibers. The spongiosa is the region of the alveolus that is enclosed between the cortical and cribriform plates. As the term *spongiosa* implies, it is composed of spongy (cancellous) bone.

13.16. B

The question requires identification of the incorrect statement. The pharyngeal tonsil is located in the nasopharynx and is therefore covered by a respiratory epithelium (pseudostratified ciliated columnar), not stratified squamous epithelium.

14
Digestive System II: Alimentary Tract

Alimentary Tract

—is composed of the tubular portion of the digestive system, namely the esophagus, stomach, small intestine, and large intestine. (See Chapter 13 for a description of the oral cavity and associated structures.)

Esophagus

—is a short muscular tube connecting the pharynx with the stomach.
—is flattened in the anteroposterior direction when empty.
—its wall is composed of four layers: the mucosa, submucosa, muscularis externa, and adventitia.

Muscularis Externa

—is unusual in that it is composed of skeletal muscle in the upper one-third, a composite of skeletal and smooth muscles in the middle one-third, and smooth muscle in the lower one-third.

Mucosa
Epithelium

—is composed of a thick, stratified, squamous nonkeratinized epithelium.

Lamina Propria

—consists of a loose connective tissue with some lymphoid infiltrates.
—also contains mucus-producing glands, known as esophageal cardiac glands.

Muscularis Mucosae

—consists of longitudinally oriented smooth muscle fibers that are especially well developed in the lower one-third of the esophagus.

Submucosa
Connective Tissue

—is dense irregular collagenous with some elastic fibers.

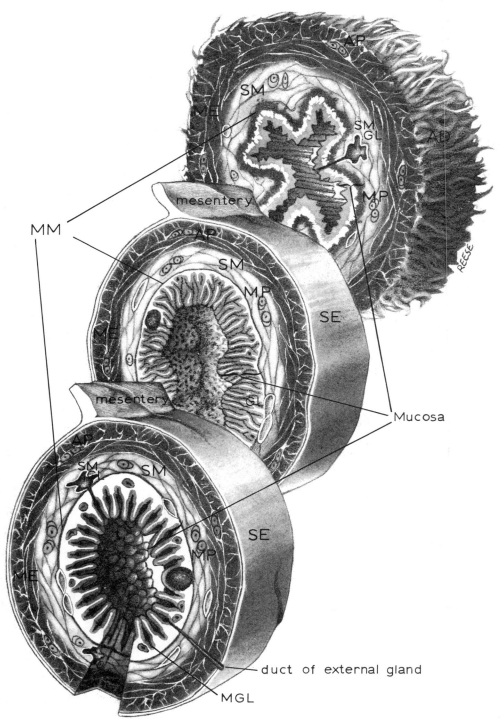

Figure 14.1. Diagrams of the general plan of the various regions of the alimentary canal: esophagus (**top**), stomach (**middle**), and small intestine (**bottom**). **MM**, muscularis mucosae. **SM**, submucosa. **ME**, muscularis externa. **AD**, adventitia. **SE**, serosa. **GL**, glands. **MGL**, mucosal glands. **MP**, Meissner's submucosal plexus. **AP**, Auerbach's myenteric plexus. (From Kelly DE, Wood RL, Enders AC: *Bailey's Textbook of Microscopic Anatomy*, ed 18. Baltimore, Williams & Wilkins, 1984.)

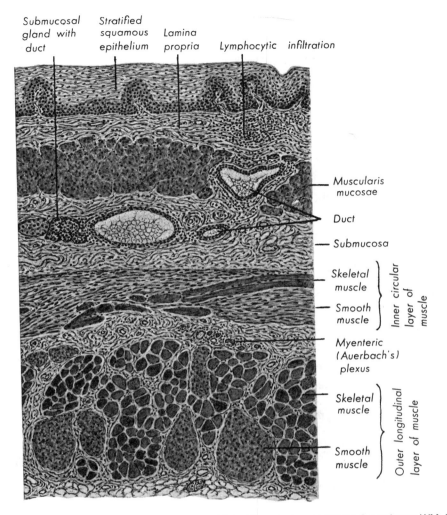

Figure 14.2. Drawing of a section of the upper one-third of the esophagus. (From Copenhaver WM, Kelly DE, Wood RL: *Bailey's Textbook of Histology*, ed 17. Baltimore, Williams & Wilkins, 1978.)

Glands

—are mucus-producing compound tubuloalveolar, known as the esophageal glands proper.

—in the alimentary tract, it is only in the esophagus and the duodenum that glands are found in the submucosa.

Innervation

—is supplied by sympathetic nerve fibers as well as parasympathetic nerve fibers derived from the vagus nerve with its associated plexus, the submucous (Meissner's) plexus.

Muscularis Externa

Inner Circular

—muscle layer is oriented as a tightly wrapped helix encircling the wall of the esophagus.

Outer Longitudinal

—layer is oriented as a loosely wrapped helix encircling the wall of the esophagus.

Muscle Type

—varies depending on the location along the esophagus.
—upper third is composed solely of skeletal muscle.
—middle third is a composite of skeletal and smooth muscles.
—lower third is composed only of smooth muscle.

Innervation

—is supplied by sympathetic fibers as well as by the vagus nerve, whose preganglionic parasympathetic fibers reach (Auerbach's) myenteric plexus, located between the inner circular and outer longitudinal layers of the muscularis externa.

Adventitia

Above the Diaphragm

—the loose connective tissue, adventitia, binds the esophagus to the surrounding structures.

Below the Diaphragm

—the adventitia is replaced by a serosa.
—difference between the serosa and adventitia is the presence of a simple squamous epithelium (mesothelium = peritoneum) covering the loose connective tissue.

Mesothelium

—provides a slippery, almost frictionless surface for organs covered by a serosa.

Histophysiology

Esophagus

—functions in conveying small portions of masticated and moistened food (bolus) from the pharynx into the stomach.
—movement of the bolus is initiated by its entry into and distension of the pharynx.
—peristaltic activity of the muscularis externa is responsible for delivering the bolus into the stomach.
—possesses two physiological sphincters, the pharyngoesophageal and the gastroesophageal, in order to ensure that the bolus will be transported in a single direction.
—these sphincters do not display histological thickening of the muscularis externa, but both evidence increased muscle tonus.

Stomach

—acidifies and converts the bolus delivered by the esophagus into a thick viscous fluid known as chyme.
—its mucosa also produces enzymes that continue digestion initiated in the oral cavity.
—is subdivided anatomically into four regions: the narrow cardia, the dome-shaped fundus, the large body, and the funnel-shaped pylorus.

Histologically

—only three regions are evident, based on the glands of the lamina propria: the cardiac, fundic, and pyloric regions.

Mucosa and Submucosa

—of the empty stomach are thrown into longitudinal folds, rugae, that disappear when the organ is distended.

Luminal Surface

—displays numerous gastric pits (foveolae), funnel-shaped invaginations of the surface epithelium, whose base receives openings of the gastric glands.
—pits are deepest in the pyloric region and shallowest in the cardiac region.

Mucosa

Epithelium

—is simple columnar, composed of mucus-producing surface lining cells.
—these are not goblet cells, and the mucus they discharge protects the lining of the stomach from autodigestion.

Lamina Propria

—is a loose connective tissue composed of a delicate network of collagenous and reticular fibers.
—contains smooth muscle cells as well as many connective tissue cells, including lymphocytes, plasma cells, mast cells, and fibroblasts.

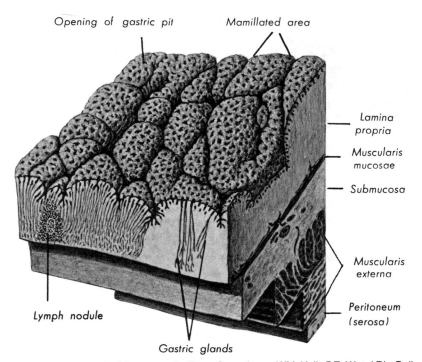

Figure 14.3. Drawing of the wall of the stomach. (From Copenhaver WM, Kelly DE, Wood RL: *Bailey's Textbook of Histology*, ed 17. Baltimore, Williams & Wilkins, 1978.)

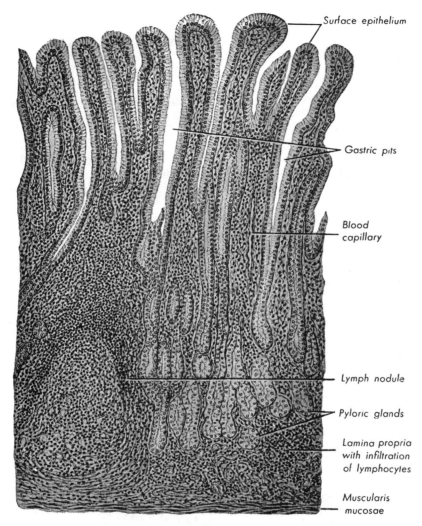

Figure 14.4. Drawing of a section of the mucosa of the pyloric stomach. (From Copenhaver WM, Kelly DE, Wood RL: *Bailey's Textbook of Histology*, ed 17. Baltimore, Williams & Wilkins, 1978.)

—also contains simple branched tubular gastric glands that are named according to their regional location (i.e., cardiac, fundic, and pyloric).

Gastric Glands

—possess an isthmus (which connects them to the bottom of a gastric pit), a neck, and a base.

—are composed of parietal (oxyntic), chief (zymogenic), mucous neck, regenerative, and APUD (amine precursor uptake and decarboxylation; also known as entero-endocrine) cells.

Fundic Glands

—contain all of these cell types, whereas both cardiac and pyloric glands lack chief cells but possess the remaining four cell types.

Parietal (oxyntic) Cells

—are pyramidal cells that secrete hydrochloric acid and gastric intrinsic factor.

—electron micrographs display a unique intracellular tubulovesicular system, a secretory canaliculus (intracellular canaliculus) lined by numerous microvilli, and many mitochondria.

—cells actively secreting hydrochloric acid display an increase in the number of microvilli and a decreased complexity of the tubulovesicular system (suggesting that the latter is a storage form of the former).

Chief (zymogenic) Cells

—are pyramidal cells located in the lower half of fundic glands.

—secrete pepsinogen, an enzyme precursor (as well as precursors of two less important enzymes, rennin and lipase).

—ultrastructural characteristics include an abundance of basally located rough endoplasmic reticulum, a supranuclearly located Golgi apparatus, and many apically located secretory (zymogen) granules.

Mucous Neck Cells

—are columnar cells, located mostly in the neck of the gland, which contain varying numbers of mucous granules.

—ultrastructural features include short microvilli, apical mucous secretory granules, a supranuclearly located Golgi apparatus, some basally located rough endoplasmic reticulum, and numerous mitochondria.

APUD (enteroendocrine) Cells

—include more than a dozen different types of cells containing (usually basally located) small granules.

—are not unusual, although with the light microscope they appear as pyramidal clear cells.

—electron micrographs display these cells as somewhat electron lucent.

—mitochondria and rough endoplasmic reticulum are well developed, and they possess a moderately developed Golgi apparatus, responsible for packaging their secretory granules.

—granules vary in size, shape, and density and contain somatostatin, secretin, serotonin, histamine, gastrin, endorphin, and cholecystokinin, among others.

—secretory products are released (by exocytosis) into the basal lamina and have a local (paracrine) effect.

—secretory products may also enter blood vessels to influence distant structures (endocrine function).

Regenerative Cells

—are narrow columnar cells responsible for replacing cells in the gland, in the pit, and on the luminal surface.

—are located mostly in the neck and isthmus regions of the gland, but some are found in the gastric pits.

Types of Glands

—cardiac, fundic, and pyloric glands are present in the stomach.

Histological Differences

—the base of the pyloric gland is much more coiled than the base of the cardiac glands.

—gastric pits in the region of the pylorus are much deeper (extend about half way into the lamina propria) than in the cardiac region (where they extend one-quarter to one-third of the way into the lamina propria).

Muscularis Mucosae

—are composed of an inner circular and an outer longitudinal layer of smooth muscle. A third layer (outermost circular) may also be present in certain regions.

Submucosa

Connective Tissue

—component is dense irregular collagenous, containing mast cells and lymphoid elements.

Neurovascular Elements

—include arterial and venous plexuses that supply and drain the vessels of the mucosa, respectively.

—submucosal plexus (of Meissner) and small lymphatic plexuses are also present.

Muscularis Externa

Inner Oblique

—smooth muscle layer is an incomplete layer, positioned just deep to the submucosa.

—is thickest in the cardia and almost absent at the lesser curvature.

Middle Circular

—smooth muscle layer is the most prominent and is continuous with the inner circular layer of the muscularis externa of the esophagus.

—becomes highly thickened at the pylorus, where it is known as the pyloric sphincter.

Outer Longitudinal

—smooth muscle layer is also incomplete. It is most developed at the cardia, the lesser and greater curvatures, and least developed at the pylorus.

Myenteric Plexus (of Auerbach)

—is located between the middle circular and outer longitudinal layers of the muscularis externa.

Serosa

—is a loose connective tissue, covered on its external surface by mesothelium.

Histophysiology

Gastric Juices

—contain water, HCl, mucus, pepsin, lipase, rennin, and electrolytes, all of which assist in digestion of food.

—low pH of the stomach (2.0) facilitates the activation of pepsinogen to pepsin, which performs its proteolytic activity at low pH environments.

Gastric Intrinsic Factor
—secreted by parietal cells, acts in the ileum to assist in the absorption of vitamin B_{12}.
—lack of gastric intrinsic factor results in pernicious anemia.

Stimulation
—of gastric secretions is due to various factors.

Hormonal
—namely gastrin (released by the APUD cells, G cells).
—gastrin release is inhibited by somatostatin (released by the APUD cells, D cells of pancreas, and small intestines).

Neural
—activity is mediated mostly by vagus nerve.

Mixing
—of the gastric contents is performed by the muscular churning actions of the three layers of the muscularis externa.

Emptying of the Stomach
—is due to peristalsis and the intermittent relaxation of the pyloric sphincter. At each relaxation a few milliliters of chyme leaves the stomach.
—rate of emptying depends on various factors, such as amount of lipids present, viscosity, osmolality, caloric density, and pH of the chyme.

Small Intestine

—positioned between the stomach and large intestine, is approximately 7 meters long.
—is composed of three histologically distinguishable regions: the duodenum, jejunum, and ileum.

Exocrine Secretions
—from the liver and pancreas as well as from the intramural glands of the small intestine contribute enzymes and other components that continue the digestive processes initiated in the oral cavity and the stomach.

Cells
—lining the lumen of the small intestine absorb the end product of digestion.
—transport end products to the lamina propria, where these materials are segregated and delivered either into the lymphatic system (fats) or into the vascular system (carbohydrates and amino acids).

Luminal Surface Modifications
—are of three types: plicae circulares, intestinal villi, and microvilli, all of which increase the surface area available for absorption.

Plicae Circulares (valves of Kerckring)
—are permanent spiral folds of the mucosa and submucosa.
—begin in the second quadrant of the duodenum and, although progressively smaller, extend as far as the first half of the ileum.
—increase the surface area by a factor of 2 to 3.

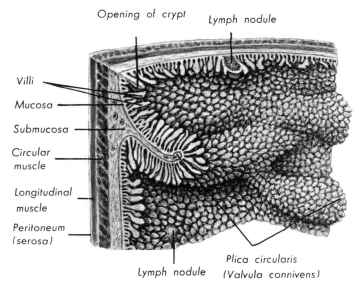

Figure 14.5. Drawing of the wall of the small intestine. (From Copenhaver WM, Kelly DE, Wood RL: *Bailey's Textbook of Histology*, ed 17. Baltimore, Williams & Wilikins, 1978.)

Intestinal Villi
—are permanent leaf or finger-like evaginations of the mucosa.
—can be as tall as 1.5 mm (in the duodenum) or as short as 0.5 mm (in the ileum).
—increase the surface area by a factor of 10.
—lamina propria of their core consists of a loose connective tissue, numerous lymphoid (especially plasma) cells, fibroblasts, smooth muscle cells, capillary loops, and a lacteal (blindly ending lymphatic channels).

Microvilli
—are located on the apical (luminal) surface of the simple columnar epithelial cells covering the villus.
—possess actin filaments that interact with the myosin filaments in the cell web, spreading the villi apart, thus increasing the surface area by an even greater extent.
—increase the surface area by a factor of about 20.

Mucosa

Epithelium
—of the small intestine is a simple columnar type composed of goblet, surface absorptive, and APUD cells.

Goblet Cells
—are unicellular glands that produce mucinogen, a substance that appears in membrane-bounded granules in the apical region of the cell.
—mucinogen accumulation distends the apical region of the cell, which is known as the theca.
—when released, mucinogen is converted to mucus, a thick, viscous substance that acts as a protective coating for the lining of the small intestine.

—the region of the cell that houses the nucleus and other organelles is the stem.

—number of goblet cells increases from the duodenum to the ileum.

—electron micrographs display some unusual globlet cells in that their mucinogen granules contain a centrally placed dense core.

Surface Absorptive Cells

—are tall columnar cells.

—free surface consists of closely packed microvilli (striated border), which have a luminal glycoprotein surface coat, the glycocalyx, composed of various enzymes.

—microvilli contain longitudinally oriented actin microfilaments that are anchored into the cell web.

—cytoplasm has numerous mitochondria, smooth and rough endoplasmic reticulum, and Golgi apparatus.

APUD (enteroendocrine) Cells

—are of varied types in the small intestine: G cells (gastrin), D cells (somatostatin), S cells (secretin), I cells (cholecystokinin), EC cells (serotonin and endorphin), and K cells (gastric inhibitory peptide), among others. (See p. 209 for a description of their structure).

Lamina Propria

—is a loose type of connective tissue forming not only the core of the villus but also the interstices between the numerous glands (crypts of Lieberkühn) of the mucosa.

—is infiltrated by lymphoid cells, possesses lymphatic nodules, blood vascular elements, smooth muscle cells, mast cells, and neural elements.

—also houses blindly ending lymphatic channels, known as lacteals, within the core of the villus.

Crypts of Lieberkühn

—are simple tubular glands that extend from the intervillous spaces to the muscularis mucosae.

—are composed of several types of epithelial cells, namely goblet cells (and oligomucous cells), columnar cells (similar to surface absorptive cells), APUD cells, regenerative cells, and Paneth cells. (Goblet, columnar, and APUD cells were described earlier; regenerative and Paneth cells are discussed next.)

Regenerative Cells

—are thin columnar stem cells.

—undergo mitotic activity to replace themselves and the various other types of epithelial cells.

—are located in the basal half of the crypts.

Paneth Cells

—are pyramidal cells located at base of the crypts of Lieberkühn.

—secrete lysozyme, an antibacterial enzyme that is contained in large, apically situated, membrane-bounded secretory granules.

—ultrastructural features include an extensive basally located rough endoplasmic reticulum, a large supranuclear Golgi apparatus, numerous mitochondria, and large, membrane-bounded, apically positioned secretory granules.

Lymphatic Nodules
—of the lamina propria are usually small and solitary in the duodenum and jejunum.
—increase in size and number in the ileum, where they form large contiguous aggregates, known as Peyer's patches, that extend through the muscularis mucosae into the submucosa.

M Cells
—specialized squamous cells, overlie the large lymphatic nodules and are believed to function in presenting antigens to macrophages and lymphocytes of the lamina propria.

Activated B Cells
—respond by forming more B cells, which, subsequent to a circuitous route, populate the lamina propria to differentiate into plasma cells.

Plasma Cells
—manufacture IgA, which will acquire an epithelially produced component to become secretory IgA.

Muscularis Mucosae
—is composed of an inner circular and an outer longitudinal layer of smooth muscle.

Submucosa
—of the small intestine is composed of fibroelastic connective tissue that contains blood and lymphatic vessels, nerves and the submucosal (Meissner's) plexus, and glands (in the duodenum).

Duodenal (Brunner's) Glands
—are located only in the submucosa of the duodenum.
—produce an alkaline, mucin-containing fluid that protects the duodenal epithelium from the acidic chyme entering from the stomach.
—also produce and release urogastrone, a polypeptide that enhances epithelial cell division and inhibits HCl production.
—may also produce a bicarbonate-rich buffering medium; however, recent investigations have not been able to confirm this.
—secretions are delivered, via ducts, into the bases of the crypts of Lieberkühn or directly into the intervillar spaces.

Muscularis Externa
—is composed of two layers of smooth muscle, an inner circular layer (which participates in the formation of the ileocecal sphincter) and an outer longitudinal layer.

Auerbach's Myenteric Plexus
—is located between the two layers of the muscularis externa.

Serosa
Adventitia and Serosa
—cover the external aspect of the duodenum.

Serosa
—covers the jejunum and ileum.

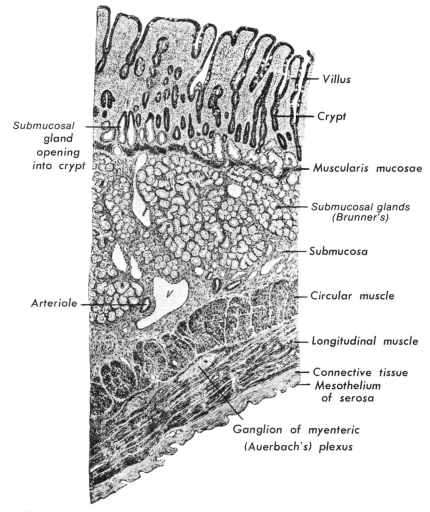

Villus

Crypt

Submucosal gland opening into crypt

Muscularis mucosae

Submucosal glands (Brunner's)

Submucosa

Arteriole

Circular muscle

Longitudinal muscle

Connective tissue
Mesothelium of serosa

Ganglion of myenteric (Auerbach's) plexus

Figure 14.6. Drawing of a section of the duodenum. (From Copenhaver WM, Kelly DE, Wood RL: *Bailey's Textbook of Histology*, ed 17. Baltimore, Williams & Wilkins, 1978.)

Large Intestine

Regions

—of the large intestine are the cecum; ascending, transverse, descending, and sigmoid colon; rectum; anal canal; and appendix.

—cecum and the various parts of the colon are histologically similar.

Mucosa of the Cecum and Colon

Mucosa

—possesses no specialized folds and lacks villi.

—is composed of an epithelium, a lamina propria (housing crypts of Lieberkühn), and a muscularis mucosae.

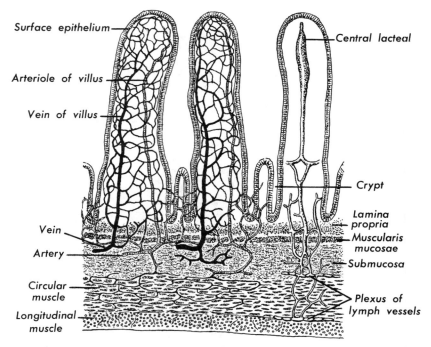

Figure 14.7. Diagram of the vascular supply and lymphatic drainage of the small intestine. (From Copenhaver WM, Kelly DE, Wood RL: *Bailey's Textbook of Histology*, ed 17. Baltimore, Williams & Wilkins, 1978.)

Epithelium

—is simple columnar with numerous goblet cells, absorptive cells, and occasional APUD (enteroendocrine) cells.

Lamina Propria

—is similar to that of the small intestine. It possesses lymphoid and vascular elements, as well as closely packed crypts of Lieberkühn.

Crypts of Lieberkühn

—possess no Paneth cells in the cecum or colon.

Muscularis Mucosae

—consists of an inner circular and an outer longitudinal layer of smooth muscle cells.

Submucosa of the Cecum and Colon

—is composed of a fibroelastic connective tissue.
—contains blood and lymphatic vessels and nerves, as well as the submucosal (Meissner's) plexus.
—glands are not present in the submucosa of this region.

Muscularis Externa of the Cecum and Colon

—is composed of an inner circular and a modified outer longitudinal layer of smooth muscle.

Longitudinal Layer

—is gathered into three flat, longitudinal ribbons of smooth muscle that form the teniae coli.

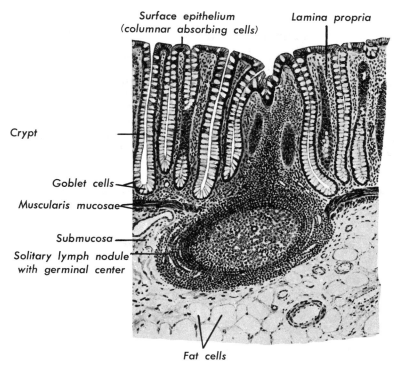

Figure 14.8. Drawing of a cross section of the colon. (From Copenhaver WM, Kelly DE, Wood RL: *Bailey's Textbook of Histology*, ed 17. Baltimore, Williams & Wilkins, 1978.)

Teniae Coli

—when continuously contracted form sacculations of the cecum and colon, known as the haustra coli.

Auerbach's (myenteric) Plexus

—is located between the two muscle layers.

Serosa and Adventitia of the Cecum and Colon

Adventitia

—covers the ascending and descending portions of the colon.

Serosa

—covers the cecum and the remainder of the colon.
—forms fat-filled outpocketings, the appendices epiploicae, that are characteristic of the colon.

Rectum

—is similar to the colon, but its crypts of Lieberkühn are fewer in number and greater in depth.

Anal Canal

—is the constricted continuation of the rectum.
—its mucosa displays longitudinal folds, the anal columns (also known as the rectal columns of Morgagni), which join each other to form anal valves.
—regions between neighboring valves are known as anal sinuses.

Epithelium

—changes from simple columnar of the rectum to simple cuboidal as far distally as the anal valves.

—distal to the anal valves it is stratified squamous nonkeratinized.

—at the anus it changes to stratified squamous keratinized (epidermis).

Lamina Propria

—is composed of fibroelastic connective tissue that contains sebaceous glands; circumanal glands, hair follicles, and large veins (which may become distended and form hemorrhoids).

Muscularis Mucosae

—consists of an inner circular and an outer longitudinal layer of smooth muscle, both of which terminate at the anal valves.

Submucosa

—is composed of dense irregular fibroelastic connective tissue. It houses large veins that may become distended, forming hemorrhoids.

Muscularis Externa

—is composed of smooth muscle. The inner circular layer forms the internal anal sphincter muscle.

Adventitia

—attaches the anus to the surrounding structures.

External Anal Sphincter

—is composed of skeletal muscle whose superficial and deep layers invest the anal canal.

—its muscle fibers are in continuous tonus, thus maintaining the anal orifice closed.

—its degree of tonus is under voluntary control, permitting restriction of the feces or defecation to occur.

Appendix

Vermiform Appendix

—is a short diverticulum arising from the blind terminus of the cecum.

—its narrow lumen is stellate or irregular in shape and often contains debris.

—its wall is usually thickened due to the presence of the almost continuous aggregates of lymphatic nodules in the mucosa and even in the submucosa (in the middle-aged individual).

Mucosa

—is lined by a simple columnar epithelium containing surface columnar and goblet cells.

—does not form villi in the appendix.

—crypts of Lieberkühn are shallow, possess some goblet cells, surface columnar cells, regenerative cells, occasional Paneth cells, and numerous (especially deep in the crypts) APUD cells.

Lamina Propria

—displays numerous lymphatic nodules (capped by M cells) and lymphoid cells.

Muscularis Mucosae

—is composed of the usual two smooth muscle layers (inner circular and outer longitudinal).

Submucosa

—is composed of fibroelastic connective tissue containing confluent lymphatic nodules and associated cell population.

—has no glands, although occasionally adipose tissue is present.

Muscularis Externa

—is composed of an inner circular and an outer longitudinal layer of smooth muscle.

Serosa

—completely surrounds the appendix.

Histophysiology

Small Intestine

Function

—digestion of foodstuffs and absorption therefrom of carbohydrates, amino acids, fats, and electrolytes.

Carbohydrates

—are hydrolyzed by salivary and pancreatic amylases into disaccharides in the lumen of the digestive tract.

—disaccharides cannot be absorbed by surface absorptive cells; therefore, disaccharidases of their glycocalyx cleave them into monosaccharides.

—monosaccharides are actively transported into the surface absorptive cells and are discharged into the lamina propria, wherefrom the vascular supply distributes them throughout the body.

Proteins

—are hydrolyzed by the various proteases within the lumen of the small intestine into small peptides and amino acids.

—small peptides and amino acids are actively transported into the surface absorptive cells, where the former are further degraded into amino acids.

Fats

—are hydrolyzed by pancreatic lipase into monoglycerides and free fatty acids and by the action of bile salts are transformed into micelles.

—products of lipid digestion then enter the surface absorptive cells.

—within the smooth endoplasmic reticulum the free fatty acids and the monoglycerides are resynthesized into triglycerides.

—in the Golgi apparatus the triglycerides are complexed with proteins to form membrane-bounded chylomicrons.

Chylomicrons

—are transported to the lateral cell membrane and released by exocytosis.

—cross the basal lamina to enter lacteals (blindly ending lymphatic capillaries of the intestinal villi) in the lamina propria.

Smooth Muscle
—contraction in the villus results in chyle being expressed into the submucosal lymphatic plexus for distribution.

Water and Electrolytes
—especially sodium and chloride are resorbed by the surface absorptive cells of the small intestine.

Large Intestine

Residual Enzymes
—transported from the small intestine, continue the digestive process in the lumen of the large intestine.

Function
—of the large intestine is to continue absorption of electrolytes and fluids, thus compacting dead bacteria and the indigestible remnants of the ingested material into feces.

Bacterial Flora
—produce vitamin B_{12} and vitamin K. The former is necessary for hemopoiesis (its absence results in pernicious anemia); the latter is a cofactor of coagulation.

Mucus
—produced by the goblet cells of the large intestine, lubricates its lining to facilitate the passage and elimination of the feces.

REVIEW TESTS
DIGESTIVE SYSTEM II

DIRECTIONS: *One* or *more* of the given completions is/are correct. Choose answer:
- A. if only **1**, **2**, and **3** are correct
- B. if only **1** and **3** are correct
- C. if only **2** and **4** are correct
- D. if only **4** is correct
- E. if **all** are correct

14.1. Stratified squamous epithelium is always present in the
1. rectum
2. jejunum
3. pyloric stomach
4. esophagus

14.2. True statements concerning the esophagus include which of the following?
1. It contains smooth muscles in its muscularis mucosae.
2. It utilizes gravitational forces to pass the bolus into the stomach.
3. It possesses skeletal muscle in its muscularis externa.
4. Its submucosa is free of glands.

14.3. Fundic glands possess the following cell type(s):
1. goblet cells
2. mucous neck cells
3. Paneth cells
4. parietal (oxyntic) cells

14.4. Substances such as secretin, cholecystokinin, and somatostatin are
1. normally secreted into the lumina of the crypts of Lieberkühn
2. enzymes utilized in digestion within the lumen of the duodenum
3. secretory products of Paneth cells
4. secretory products of APUD (enteroendocrine) cells

14.5. Luminal surface modifications of the duodenum and jejunum include
1. microvilli
2. villi
3. plicae circulares
4. rugae

14.6. True statements concerning the ileum include the following:
1. The mucosa of the ileum houses few goblet cells.
2. Lacteals of the lamina propria collect only carbohydrates and amino acids.
3. The submucosa houses seromucous glands.
4. Lymphatic nodules are prevalent in the lamina propria.

14.7. Absorption of electrolytes and water are functions performed mostly by the
1. esophagus
2. stomach
3. appendix
4. colon

221

DIRECTIONS The following questions or statements refer to the photomicrograph (Fig. 14.9). The letters on the figures are answers to the numbered items appearing below the photomicrograph. For each numbered item, select the *one* letter that *best* corresponds to that item. Each letter may be used once, more than once, or not at all.

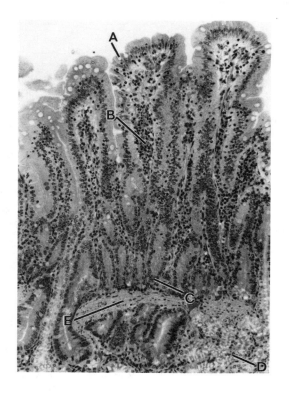

Figure 14.9.

14.8. goblet cell

14.9. lamina propria

14.10. muscularis mucosae

14.11. location of lacteals

14.12. location of Paneth cells

14.13. separates the lamina propria from the submucosa

ANSWERS AND EXPLANATIONS

DIGESTIVE SYSTEM II

14.1. D (4)
The rectum, jejunum, and the pyloric stomach are lined by simple columnar epithelia. With the exception of regions of the anus all of the alimentary tract distal to the esophagus is lined by simple columnar epithelium.

14.2. B (1 and 3)
The esophagus is unusual in that it possesses a combination of smooth and skeletal muscles in its muscularis externa: the proximal third is completely skeletal, the middle third is a combination of smooth and skeletal, whereas the distal third is composed completely of smooth muscle. These muscles propel the bolus into the stomach by the use of peristaltic movement. The muscularis mucosae, however, is composed only of smooth muscle. Finally, the esophagus and the duodenum are the only two regions of the alimentary tract that possess glands in their submucosa.

14.3. C (2 and 4)
Goblet cells and Paneth cells are not found in the stomach. Goblet cells are found only distal to the stomach, whereas Paneth cells are present in the base of the crypts of Lieberkühn.

14.4. D (4)
Secretin, cholecystokinin, and somatostatin are paracrine hormones. They are not secreted into the lumen of the digestive tract. Paneth cells produce an antibacterial agent, lysozyme.

14.5. A (1, 2, and 3)
Rugae are surface modifications of the empty stomach that disappear upon distension of that organ.

14.6. D (4)
The number of goblet cells increases as one progresses distal to the duodenum. Lacteals are blindly ending lymphatic channels that collect lipids. Only the submucosae of the esophagus and the duodenum possess glands.

14.7. D (4)
Very little absorption occurs in the esophagus and the stomach. The appendix, most probably, does not function in absorption. It is the function of the large intestine to absorb fluids and electrolytes.

For questions **14.8** to **14.13**, refer to Figure 14.9, a section of the jejunum.

14.8. A, goblet cell

14.9. B, lamina propria

14.10. E, muscularis mucosae

14.11. B, location of lacteals

14.12. C, location of Paneth cells

14.13. E, separates the lamina propria from the submucosa

15
Digestive System III: Glands

Extrinsic Glands

—of the digestive system are located outside the wall of the alimentary canal and deliver their secretion into the lumen via a system of ducts.

—provide enzymes, buffers, emulsifiers, and lubricants for the digestive tract, as well as hormones, proteins, globulins, and numerous additional products for the remainder of the body.

—are the salivary glands (parotid, sublingual, and submandibular), the pancreas, and the liver.

Major Salivary Glands

Parotid Gland

Classification

—purely serous, compound, tubuloalveolar gland.

Capsule

—formed by the continuation of the superficial cervical fascia, is mostly collagenous in nature.

—forms broad bands of trabeculae (septa) that subdivide the gland into lobes and lobules.

Trabeculae

—convey blood and lymph vessels, ducts, and nerves into the substance of the gland.

—often contain fat cells in older individuals.

Acini

—although are said to be composed of purely serous cells, they are actually seromucous in character.

—are surrounded by myoepithelial cells.

—their center contains the lumen.

Acinar Cells

—pyramidal cells, whose apical aspects usually contain secretory granules.

—nucleus is round and basally located.

—cytoplasm contains extensive rough endoplasmic reticulum, a well-developed Golgi apparatus, and numerous mitochondria.

Myoepithelial Cells

—are stellate shaped.
—their cytoplasm is difficult to discern with the light microscope.
—electron micrographs demonstrate that they resemble smooth muscle cells and are contractile.

Ducts

—are of various diameters.

Stensen's Duct

—is the largest (main parotid duct).
—opens into the oral vestibule at the parotid papilla.
—is lined by a simple columnar or pseudostratified epithelium.

Striated Ducts

—are lined by high cuboidal cells.
—have basal striations that parallel the longitudinal axis of the cell.
—striations are due to deep infoldings of the basal plasma membrane, which compartmentalize mitochondria.

Intercalated Ducts

—are the smallest ducts.
—are lined by a simple cuboidal epithelium and lie interposed among the acini, where they constitute the initial part of the duct system.

Sublingual Gland

Classification

—mixed, compound, tubuloalveolar gland.

Capsule

—see preceding discussion of parotid gland.

Acini

—are mostly mucous but capped with serous demilunes. Occasionally, purely mucous acini are present, but purely serous units are not present.

Acinar Cells

—the mucous cells are pyramidal shaped, with their nuclei flattened against the basal plasma membrane.
—light micrographs display pale blue cells with a "frothy" appearance (with hematoxylin and eosin).
—electron micrographs demonstrate that the apical region of the cell contains a large number of mucinogen granules.
—organelles of the cell (Golgi apparatus, rough endoplasmic reticulum, and mitochondria) are located between the granules and the nucleus.

Serous Demilune Cells

—are located peripheral to the mucous acini and deliver their secretions into intercellular spaces between the neighboring mucus-producing cells.

Myoepithelial Cells

—see preceding discussion of parotid gland.

Ducts

—short intercalated and striated ducts are present, but are few in number.

Submandibular Gland

Classification

—mixed, compound tubuloalveolar gland.

Capsule

—see preceding discussions of parotid and sublingual glands.

Acini

—composed mostly of serous acini; however, groups of mucous acini with serous demilunes are also present.

Acinar Cells

—see discussions of parotid and sublingual glands.

Myoepithelial Cells

—see discussions of parotid and sublingual glands.

Ducts

—intercalated ducts are short, but present; striated ducts are long and clearly evident.

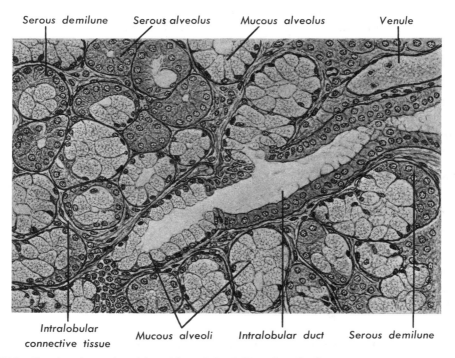

Figure 15.1. Drawing of a section of the sublingual gland. (From Copenhaver WM, Kelly DE, Wood RL: *Bailey's Textbook of Histology*, ed 17. Baltimore, Williams & Wilkins, 1978.)

Saliva

Volume
—average daily production is 1.0 to 1.2 liters.

Function
—protects the oral cavity by lubrication, control of bacterial flora (by the presence of lysozyme, lactoferrin, and IgA), and its cleansing action.
—assists in taste sensation.
—initiates digestion of carbohydrates via action of its enzyme, salivary amylase.

Primary Secretion
—saliva secreted by the acini, prior to modification by the system of ducts, resembles extracellular fluid.

Final Secretion
—intercalated ducts may deliver bicarbonate ions into the saliva.
—striated ducts (via their sodium pump) remove sodium and chloride ions from the luminal fluid and actively pump potassium ions into it.

Saliva
—is a hypotonic solution.

Pancreas

—is a retroperitoneal gland that produces both exocrine and endocrine secretions.
—is subdivided into the following regions: head, uncinate process, neck, body, and tail. Tail contains the highest concentration of endocrine tissue (islets of Langerhans).

Capsule
—is composed of delicate connective tissue that subdivides the gland into lobules by forming numerous septa. Septa convey blood and lymph vessels, nerves, and ducts in and out of the gland.

Exocrine Pancreas

Classification
—a purely serous, compound tubuloalveolar gland.

Acini
—only serous, whose centers contain centroacinar cells, which form the beginning of the duct system in the pancreas.

Intercellular Canaliculi
—lead from between acinar cells to the lumen of the acinus.

Acinar Cells
—are pyramidal in shape and have a round nucleus that is basally located.
—basal region is strongly basophilic.
—apical region is densely packed with secretory granules (zymogen granules).

—electron micrographs demonstrate abundant rough endoplasmic reticulum, an extensive Golgi apparatus, numerous mitochondria, and many free ribosomes.

—secretory granules are all membrane bound and are occasionally noted to be in the process of being released in "chains" that extend to the lumen of the acinus.

Myoepithelial Cells

—are not present in the pancreas.

Ducts

—extend from within the acini.

Centroacinar Cells

—are low cuboidal in shape, and they constitute the initial part of the intercalated duct.

Intercalated Ducts

—lead into a small number of intralobular ducts, which in turn empty into the large interlobular ducts.

Interlobular Ducts

—are located between lobules in extensive connective tissue and empty into the main (or accessory) pancreatic duct.

Pancreatic Duct

—the main pancreatic duct, delivers the pancreatic secretions into the duodenum at the papilla of Vater.

Histophysiology

—two hormones, released by APUD cells of the digestive tract, control the release of pancreatic secretions.

Cholecystokinin (pancreozymin)

—induces the acinar cells to release pancreatic juices rich in digestive enzymes.

—the enzymes are trypsin, chymotrypsin, peptidase, pancreatic amylase and lipase, and ribo- and deoxyribonucleases.

Secretin

—induces the intercalated ducts to secrete large quantities of an enzyme-poor, alkaline fluid that probably functions in neutralizing the acidic chyme that enters the duodenum.

Endocrine Pancreas

Islets of Langerhans

—are spherical clumps of richly vascularized endocrine cells.

—lie scattered in an apparently random fashion among the acini of the exocrine pancreas.

—are more numerous in the tail region.

—are composed of several cell types having different functions.

Cells

—are indistinguishable in routinely stained sections but can be differentiated by the use of special stains.

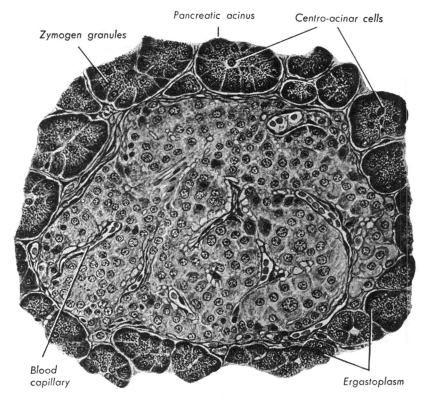

Zymogen granules

Pancreatic acinus

Centro-acinar cells

Blood capillary

Ergastoplasm

Figure 15.2. Drawing of a section of the pancreas displaying an islet of Langerhans. (From Copenhaver WM, Kelly DE, Wood RL: *Bailey's Textbook of Histology*, ed 17. Baltimore, Williams & Wilkins, 1978.)

Alpha Cells

—are preferentially positioned at the islet's periphery.

—electron micrographs demonstrate that alpha cells have spherical, membrane-bound, electron-dense granules.

Beta Cells

—constitute the majority and occupy mostly the center of each islet.

Granules

—are also membrane bound but are smaller than those of alpha cells.

—are characterized by the presence of an irregular dense core, surrounded by an electron-lucent periphery.

Delta$_1$ Cells

—less common than the other two and may be recognized in the electron microscope by their relatively large, electron-lucent granules.

—granules, whose membranes are usually not well defined.

Other Cell Types

—include C, E, G, and PP cells.

Histophysiology
—each cell type produces a specific hormone:
—alpha cells manufacture glucagon (elevates blood glucose levels).
—beta cells produce insulin (lowers blood glucose levels).
—delta$_1$ cells manufacture somatostatin (a hormone that controls the release of insulin and glucagon, thus possibly reducing the volume of alkaline-rich pancreatic juices).
—C cells may represent immature or degranulated islet cells.
—PP cells apparently release pancreatic polypeptide, a hormone that may act to reduce the release of both enzyme-rich and alkaline-rich pancreatic secretions.
—G cells release gastrin, a hormone that functions in modulating the release of HCl by the parietal cells of the stomach.

Liver
—is the second largest organ in the body.
—is composed of a single type of parenchymal cell, the hepatocyte.

Hepatocyte
—possesses a myriad of both endocrine and exocrine functions.

Glisson's Capsule
—is composed of thin connective tissue that subdivides the liver into lobes and lobules.

Blood Supply
—of the liver is derived from two sources: abdominal aorta, via the hepatic artery; portal vein, which brings nutrient-laden blood from the alimentary tract and the spleen.

Porta Hepatis
—is the region where the hepatic artery and the portal vein enter and the hepatic ducts leave the liver.

Drainage
—of blood is via the hepatic vein.
—hepatic vein is formed by the union of numerous sublobular veins.
—sublobular veins collect blood from the central vein of each classical liver lobule.

Bile
—leaves the liver via the hepatic ducts.
—is delivered to the gallbladder.

Liver Lobules
—there are three types of liver lobules: classical (hexagonal in histologic section); portal lobule (triangular in histologic section); liver acinus of Rappaport (liver acinus; diamond shaped in histologic section).

Classical Lobule
—is based on the pig's liver, where connective tissue elements clearly delineate it.
—portal area (portal canal; triad) is present at each corner of the lobule.
—portal area contains branches of the portal vein, hepatic artery, bile duct, and lymph vessel.

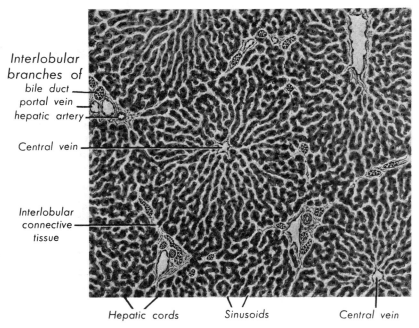

Interlobular branches of
bile duct
portal vein
hepatic artery

Central vein

Interlobular connective tissue

Hepatic cords   Sinusoids   Central vein

Figure 15.3. Drawing of a section of the liver. (From Copenhaver WM, Kelly DE, Wood RL: *Bailey's Textbook of Histology*, ed 17. Baltimore, Williams & Wilkins, 1978.)

Plates of Hepatocytes
—compose the bulk of the lobule.
—are arranged in a radial fashion, radiating from the region of a central vein.
—blood flows from the periphery of the lobule toward the central vein.

Bile
—the exocrine secretion of the liver, flows through bile canaliculi.

Bile Canaliculi
—are slender intercellular spaces between neighboring hepatocytes.
—convey bile to canals of Hering.
—canals of Hering deliver bile to bile ducts in the portal area at the periphery of the classical lobule.
—flow of bile and blood occurs in opposite directions.

Sinusoids
—are endothelial lined spaces between neighboring plates of hepatocytes.
—receive blood from the vessels in the portal area and deliver it to the central vein.

Endothelial Cells
—lining sinusoids have large fenestrations and also display discontinuities between neighboring cells.

Kupffer Cells
—are also present within the endothelial lining.
—are phagocytic cells that are derived from monocytes.

Space of Disse

—is visualized by electron microscopy as a subendothelial space between the liver cells and the lining cells of the sinusoids.

Contains

—stellate-shaped fat storing cells (which preferentially store vitamin A).
—reticular fibers (which maintain the architecture of the sinusoids).
—nonmyelinated nerve fibers.
—short, blunt microvilli of hepatocytes.

Functions

—in the exchange of material between the bloodstream and the hepatocytes (which do not contact the bloodstream).

Basal Lamina

—is not present in this space.

Portal Lobule

—is based on the liver's exocrine function. In many exocrine glands, the duct is in the center of a lobule.
—is a triangular region whose three apices are neighboring central veins, selected in such a fashion that the triangle thus constructed will have a portal area in its center.

Liver Acinus (of Rappaport)

—is another interpretation of lobulation in the liver.
—is based on blood flow.
—is a diamond-shaped structure, envisioned as the amalgamation of two equilateral triangular areas derived from two adjoining classical lobules, where the bases of the two triangles parallel each other.
—apices include the central vein of the first classical lobule, the two adjoining portal areas that are shared by the two neighboring classical lobules, and the central vein of the second classical lobule.

Zonation

—blood enters the sinusoids from vessels located in the interface between the two neighboring classical lobules (the bases of the equilateral triangles).

Hepatocytes

—in the vicinity of this interface are the first to be "exposed" to the entering blood.
—nearer the central vein are the last to be "exposed."

Three Zones

—exist within each liver acinus of Rappaport: first in the immediate vicinity of the blood supply, third in the area of the central vein, and second in between these two areas.

Hepatocytes

—are large, polyhedral cells that stain light pink with hematoxylin and eosin.
—usually possess one (or two), centrally placed (occasionally enlarged polyploid) round nucleus.
—frequently more than two nuclei may be present in a single cell.
—bile canaliculi are evident between neighboring hepatocytes.

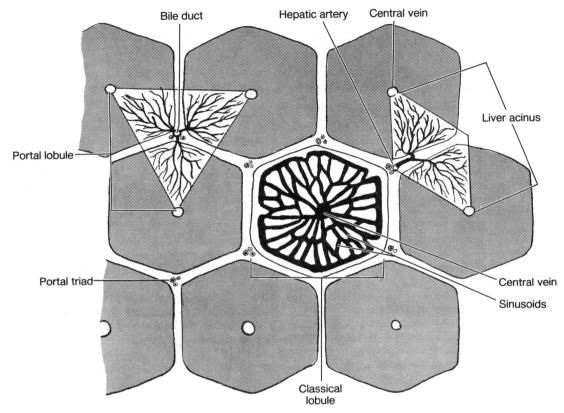

Figure 15.4. Diagram illustrating lobulation in the liver. (From Krause WJ, Cutts JH: *Concise Text of Histology*, ed 2. Baltimore, Williams & Wilkins, 1986.)

Electron Micrographs

—demonstrate that these cells are rich in rough and smooth endoplasmic reticula and mitochondria and possess several Golgi regions.

—demonstrate that both lysosomes and peroxisomes are well represented.

—lipid droplets and glycogen are also abundant.

Surfaces

—are of two types: those that border the space of Disse; those that are adjacent neighboring hepatocytes.

Adjacent Space of Disse

—microvilli assist in the transfer of materials to and from hepatocytes. It is here that the endocrine secretions of the liver also take place.

Adjacent Neighboring Hepatocytes

—form small, tunnel-like bile canaliculi that represent intercellular spaces.

—form occluding junctions at each surface of the bile canaliculus.

Microvilli

—extend into the bile canaliculus from each hepatocyte.

Bile Canaliculi

—receive the exocrine secretion of the liver (bile), thus representing the beginning of the duct system.

Gap Junctions

—are also formed where neighboring hepatocytes contact one another.

Intrahepatic Bile Ducts

—consist of the bile canaliculi; cholangioles; canals of Hering (bile ductules), lined by a layer of low cuboidal cells; and bile ducts, lined by a single layer of cuboidal cells.

Extrahepatic Bile Ducts

—receive bile from the main ducts of the liver. The major ducts are the right and left hepatic ducts.

Hepatic Ducts

—join to form the common hepatic duct.

Cystic Duct

—in common with the common hepatic duct forms the common bile duct.
—leads to the gallbladder.

Common Bile Duct

—(frequently in common with the main pancreatic duct) delivers its contents into the lumen of the duodenum via the papilla of Vater (duodenal papilla).

Sphincter of Oddi

—is proximal to the papilla of Vater.
—is formed by smooth muscle in the wall of the common bile duct.
—directs the flow of bile into the gallbladder or into the lumen of the duodenum.

Histophysiology of Liver

—although the liver performs a myriad of different functions, every hepatocyte is capable of accomplishing each task.

Exocrine Function

—the production of bile.

Bile

—is composed of bilirubin, bile acids, cholesterol, phospholipids, ions, and water.

Endocrine Secretions

—include glucose as well as several plasma proteins (such as prothrombin, fibrinogen, albumin, Factor III, and very-low-density lipoproteins).

Storage Functions

—carbohydrates (in the form of glycogen) and lipids are stored in hepatocytes.

Gluconeogenesis

—another function, is the process whereby amino acids and lipids are converted into glucose.

Detoxification

—is another function, whereby the liver detoxifies various drugs and toxins.

Phagocytosis

—is a process performed by Kupffer cells, which remove debris and cellular fragments from the bloodstream.

IgA Uptake

—from the bloodstream occurs at the space of Disse.

—IgA is released into the bile canaliculi for eventual transport into the intestine, where it serves a protective function.

Gallbladder

—is a small, pear-shaped organ.

—stores and concentrates bile manufactured by the liver.

—storage volume is approximately 40 to 60 ml.

—muscular wall contracts to force the bile in its lumen into the duodenum, where the bile acts to emulsify fats.

—contraction is facilitated by the hormone cholecystokinin.

—has a relatively simple structure, composed of a mucosa, smooth muscle layer, dense collagenous connective tissue, and a serosa.

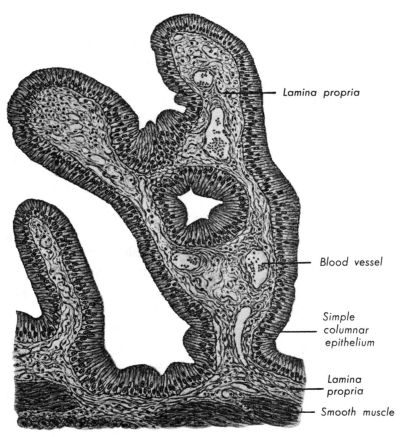

Figure 15.5. Diagram of a section of the gallbladder. (From Copenhaver WM, Bunge RP, Bunge MB: *Bailey's Textbook of Histology*, ed 16. Baltimore, Williams & Wilkins, 1971.)

Mucosa

—is composed of a simple columnar epithelium and a richly vascularized lamina propria.

Lamina Propria

—presents a highly convoluted architecture in the empty gallbladder. Proximal to the cystic duct, the lamina propria displays simple tubuloalveolar mucous glands.

Muscle Layer

—is composed of a thin layer of smooth muscle cells, oriented in an oblique fashion.

Connective Tissue

—is dense, irregular collagenous, housing nerves and blood vessels.

Serosa

—the peritoneum covers most of the gallbladder, except where the organ is attached to the liver.

Other Features

—sinuses of Rokitansky-Aschoff are deep invaginations of the epithelium that may extend into the perimuscular connective tissue layer.

—ducts of Luschka are nonfunctional, blind-ending ducts in the vicinity of the neck of the gallbladder.

REVIEW TESTS
DIGESTIVE SYSTEM III

DIRECTIONS: *One* or *more* of the given completions or answers is/are correct. Choose answer:

A. if only **1**, **2**, and **3** are correct
B. if only **1** and **3** are correct
C. if only **2** and **4** are correct
D. if only **4** is correct
E. if **all** are correct

15.1. Myoepithelial cells are found in the following glands:
1. parotid
2. submandibular
3. sublingual
4. pancreas

15.2. Serous demilunes are present in the following glands:
1. sublingual
2. pancreas
3. submandibular
4. parotid

15.3. Longitudinally arrayed mitochondria are located in the basal infoldings of
1. interlobar ducts
2. interlobular ducts
3. intercalated ducts
4. striated ducts

15.4. Saliva
1. performs in antibacterial activities
2. is the equivalent of the primary secretion
3. contains IgA
4. initiates the digestion of proteins

15.5. Centroacinar cells of the exocrine pancreas
1. belong to the intercalated system of ducts
2. belong to the striated system of ducts
3. are affected by the hormone secretin
4. are affected by the hormone cholecystokinin

15.6. The pancreas, a gland that produces both exocrine and endocrine secretory products,
1. possesses islets of Langerhans
2. displays round nuclei in its acinar cells
3. has more beta cells than alpha cells
4. exhibits large, electron-lucent granules in its D cells

15.7. The portal area of the liver houses
1. branches of the hepatic vein
2. branches of the portal vein
3. canals of Hering
4. lymphatic vessels

15.8. Liver sinusoids
1. are continuous with bile canaliculi
2. are surrounded by a well-developed basal lamina
3. are lined by nonfenestrated endothelial cells
4. deliver blood to the central vein

15.9. Hepatocytes are large polyhedral cells that
1. are rich in glycogen granules
2. manufacture several blood proteins
3. possess endocrine functions
4. possess exocrine functions

15.10. The liver acinus of Rappaport
1. is synonymous with the portal lobule
2. is based on the flow of bile
3. follows the contours of Glisson's capsule
4. bears a relationship to blood flow

DIRECTIONS: The following terms refer to the electron micrograph of two liver cells (Fig. 15.6). The letters on the figure are answers to the numbered items appearing below the photomicrograph. For each numbered item select the *one* letter that *best* corresponds to that item. Each letter may be used once, more than once, or not at all.

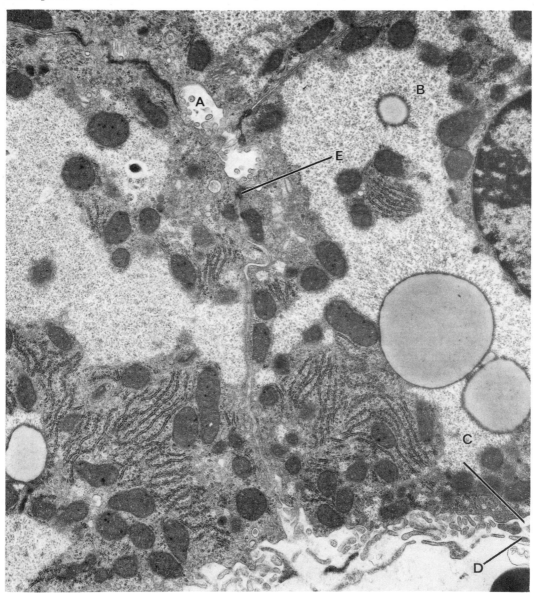

Figure 15.6. From Gartner LP, Hiatt JL: *Atlas of Histology*. Baltimore, Williams & Wilkins, 1987.

15.11. bile canaliculus

15.12. sinusoidal lining cell

15.13. glycogen deposits

15.14. space of Disse

15.15. occluding junction

DIRECTIONS: The following terms refer to the photomicrograph (Fig. 15.7). The letters on the figure are answers to the numbered items appearing below the photomicrograph. For each numbered item select the *one* letter that *best* corresponds to that item. Each letter may be used once, more than once, or not at all.

Figure 15.7. From Gartner LP, Hiatt JL: *Atlas of Histology*. Baltimore, Williams & Wilkins, 1987.

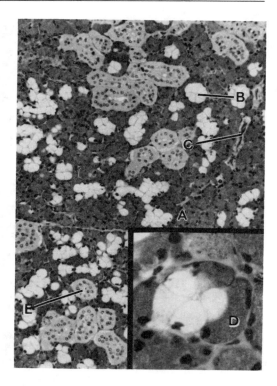

15.16. intercalated duct

15.17. serous acinus

15.18. serous demilune

15.19. mucous acinus

15.20. connective tissue septum

ANSWERS AND EXPLANATIONS

DIGESTIVE SYSTEM III

15.1. A (1, 2, and 3)
Myoepithelial cells are smooth muscle-like cells that are located at the periphery of the acini of certain glands. These cells always surround acini of the major salivary glands but not those of the pancreas.

15.2. B (1 and 3)
Serous demilunes are collections of cells, manufacturing a serous secretion, which are located at the periphery of mucous acini. Therefore, they are found only in glands that produce a mixed type of secretion.

15.3. D (4)
Striated ducts are lined by high cuboidal cells that demonstrate basal striations parallel to the longitudinal axis of the cells. These striations are due to compartmentalized mitochondria that lie within deep infoldings of the basal plasma membrane.

15.4. B (1 and 3)
Saliva (manufactured by the three major and numerous minor salivary glands) contains lysozyme, an enzyme that possesses antimicrobial activity. Moreover, IgA (immunoglobulin A) is also secreted into the saliva. Salivary amylase, also present in saliva, initiates the digestion of carbohydrates, not proteins. Primary secretion, the product that is released by the cells of the acinus, becomes modified by cells of the intercalated and striated ducts.

15.5. B (1 and 3)
The intercalated system of ducts of the pancreas begins within the acinus as centroacinar cells. The hormone secretin, released by APUD cells of the digestive tract (small intestine), stimulates the intercalated ducts to form and release an alkaline-rich pancreatic secretion. The hormone cholecystokinin (also formed by APUD cells of the small intestine) stimulates the release of the enzyme-rich secretions (zymogen granules) manufactured by the acinar cells.

15.6. E (all are correct)

15.7. C (2 and 4)
Branches of the portal vein, lymphatic vessels, bile ducts, and hepatic artery are located in the connective tissue space known as the portal area. Canals of Hering are situated in the interfaces between classical lobules and are tributaries of bile ducts that are positioned in the portal area. The only branch of the hepatic vein located within hepatic lobules is the central vein, which does not reside in the portal area.

15.8. D (4)
Liver sinusoids, fenestrated endothelial cell–lined vascular channels, deliver their blood directly into the central vein. Unlike other blood vessels, their endothelial cells do not lie upon a basal lamina. Bile canaliculi are intercellular spaces between adjacent liver cells that lead to the periphery of the classical lobule, where they deliver their contents, bile, into cholangioles, thence into the canals of Hering and small bile ducts.

15.9. E (all are correct)

15.10. D (4)
The liver acinus of Rappaport is an interpretation of liver lobulation based on the flow of blood from the vessels leading directly into the sinusoids. The availability of nutrients and additional bloodborne materials to hepatocytes in fixed locations determines the definition of this liver lobule. The acinus is subdivided into three regions as a function of distance from the source of blood supply. The portal lobule is based on the flow of bile, not on blood flow. Connective tissue, derived from Glisson's capsule, subdivides the liver into lobe and lobules. The latter is especially prominent in the pig, camel, and certain other mammals, but much less prominent in the human.

For **15.11** to **15.15**, refer to Figure 15.6, an electron micrograph of two liver cells.

15.11. **A**, bile canaliculus

15.12. **D**, sinusoidal lining cell

15.13. **B**, glycogen deposits

15.14. **C**, space of Disse

15.15. **E**, occluding junction

15.16. **E**, intercalated duct

15.17. **A**, serous acinus

15.18. **D**, serous demilune

15.19. **B**, mucous acinus

15.20. **C**, connective tissue septum

For **15.16** to **15.20**, refer to Figure 15.7, a section of the submandibular gland.

16
Urinary System

Urinary System

—includes the kidneys, ureters, urinary bladder, and urethra, all of which function in excretion.
—functions to clear the blood of waste products and regulate the concentration of body fluids.
—kidney also produces the hormone erythropoietin (which stimulates erythrocyte production) and the enzyme renin (which influences blood pressure and the concentration of sodium in the body fluids).

Kidneys

Macroscopic Features

Location
—paired, bean-shaped organs situated retroperitoneally against the posterior abdominal wall.

Hilus
—a concavity on the medial border of the kidney where arteries, veins, lymphatics, nerves, and the renal pelvis are present. The hilus is continuous with the renal sinus (a central cavity containing fat).

Renal Pelvis
—funnel-shaped expansion of the upper end of the ureter.
—is continuous with the major calyces, which in turn subdivide into minor calyces.

Cortex and Medulla
—easily identified in a hemisected kidney.
—cortex appears granular and is located superficially.
—medulla appears striated and lies deeper.
—renal corpuscles and convoluted tubules comprise most of the cortex, while the medulla is composed of several renal pyramids.
—at the apex of each renal pyramid is the renal papilla with its perforated tip (area cribrosa), which projects into the lumen of a minor calyx.
—cortical tissue, the renal columns of Bertin, extend between adjacent renal pyramids.

Renal Lobe
—consists of a renal pyramid together with its closely associated cortical tissue.

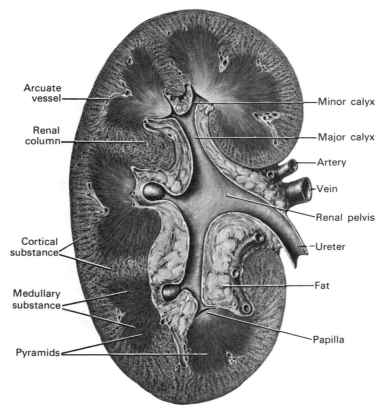

Figure 16.1. Diagram of a longitudinal section of the kidney. (From Kelly DE, Wood RL, Enders AC: *Bailey's Textbook of Microscopic Anatomy*, ed 18. Baltimore, Williams & Wilkins, 1984.)

Medullary Ray

—is a group of straight tubules that project into the cortex from the base of each renal pyramid.

Renal Lobule

—consists of a medullary ray (at its center) and the closely associated cortical tissue surrounding it.

—all nephrons in a single lobule are drained by the same collecting tubule.

Uriniferous Tubule

Components

—two principal parts, the nephron and the collecting tubule.

—each originates from separate primordia in the embryo.

Nephron

—includes the renal corpuscle, proximal convoluted tubule, descending pars recta (straight portion) of proximal tubule, thin segment, ascending thick limb (of the distal tubule), and distal convoluted tubule.

—may be classified as cortical or juxtamedullary, depending on location of the renal corpuscle.

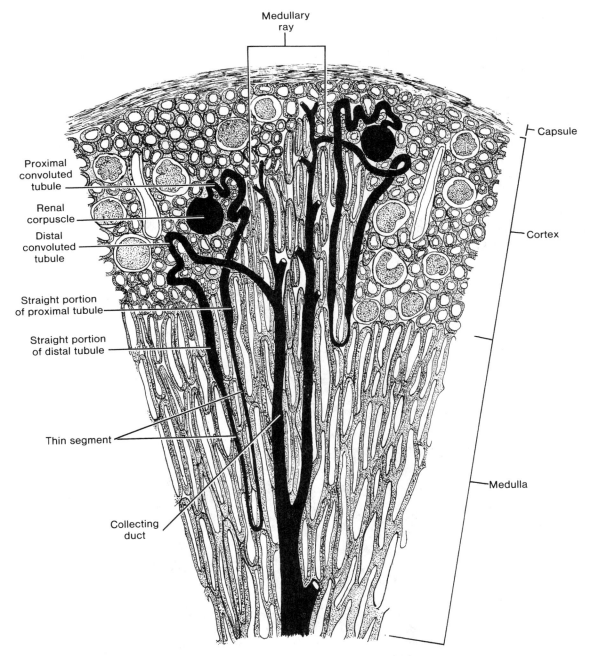

Figure 16.2. Diagram of the uriniferous tubules. (From Krause WJ, Cutts JH: *Concise Text of Histology*, ed 2. Baltimore, Williams & Wilkins, 1986.)

—cortical nephrons usually possess short loops of Henle in contrast to juxtamedullary nephrons.

—long loops of Henle, which extend deep into the medulla, are responsible for establishing (by a countercurrent mechanism) the interstitial concentration gradient that enables the kidney to form hypertonic urine.

Renal Corpuscle

—includes two parts, the glomerulus (a capillary tuft) and Bowman's capsule.
—simple squamous epithelium that composes the outer wall of Bowman's capsule is known as the parietal layer (capsular epithelium).
—modified simple squamous epithelial layer investing the glomerular capillaries is referred to as the visceral layer (glomerular epithelium).
—Bowman's space (capsular space) is the narrow chalice-shaped cavity between the visceral and parietal epithelial layers.
—at the vascular pole the afferent glomerular arteriole enters and the efferent glomerular arteriole leaves the glomerulus.
—at the urinary pole the capsular space becomes continuous with the lumen of the proximal convoluted tubule.

Podocytes

—are modified simple squamous epithelial cells comprising the visceral layer (glomerular epithelium).
—appear stellate and unusual in shape.

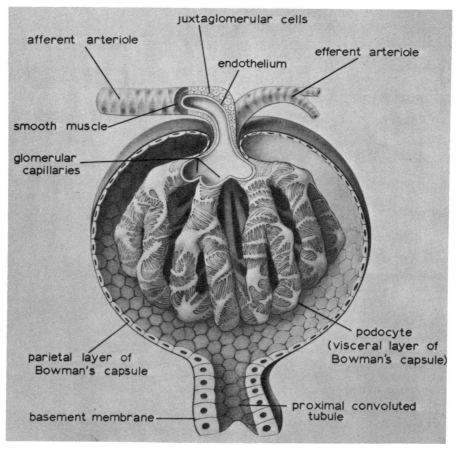

Figure 16.3. Diagram of a renal corpuscle. (From Kelly DE, Wood RL, Enders AC: *Bailey's Textbook of Microscopic Anatomy*, ed 18. Baltimore, Williams & Wilkins, 1984.)

—have several radiating primary processes that give rise to many secondary processes (pedicels; foot processes).

—pedicels interdigitate with similar processes from adjacent podocytes.

—between adjacent pedicels are filtration slits, 20 to 30 nm in width (slit pores), that are bridged by a layer of filamentous material referred to as a slit diaphragm (membrane).

—pedicel surface facing Bowman's space has a protein coating (podocalyxin) that stains with cationic dyes and is believed to maintain the organization and shape of these processes.

Basal Lamina

—associated with the filtration barrier is unusually thick (0.1 to 0.15 μm).

—is located between the podocytes and the endothelial cells in the glomerulus.

—has three distinct zones: the lamina rara externa (an electron-lucent area adjacent to the epithelium), the lamina rara interna (an electron-lucent region adjacent to the capillary endothelium), and the lamina densa (a thicker amorphous intermediate zone that appears more electron dense).

Endothelium

—lining the capillaries is thin and fenestrated.

—has no diaphragms extending across its large fenestrae (60 to 90 nm diameter).

—contains most organelles in the thicker regions of unfenestrated cytoplasm.

Filtration Barrier

—functions to filter the blood plasma and is located in the renal corpuscle.

—permits water, ions, and small molecules (ultrafiltrate) to enter the capsular space.

—prohibits protein molecules with a molecular weight greater than 69,000 or molecules with a high net negative charge from entering the capsular space.

—components of the barrier include the fenestrated endothelium, the basal lamina, and the filtration slits (with diaphragms) between pedicels.

—current studies indicate that the glomerular basal lamina is responsible for filtration selectivity, which depends not only on the size but also on the shape and charge of the molecule.

Mesangium

—comprises the interstitial spaces of the glomerulus between the capillaries.

—contains mesangial cells and extracellular matrix material.

—is the area where phagocytic mesangial cells help maintain functional integrity of the basal lamina in the filtration barrier by phagocytosing large protein molecules and/or debris.

—mesangial cells also contract to decrease surface area available for filtration, and they have receptors for angiotensin II and atrial natriuretic factor.

Proximal Convoluted Tubule

—leaves urinary pole of the renal corpuscle.

—is the longest segment of the nephron, lined by a single layer of pyramidal-shaped cells that have a well-developed brush border (microvilli).

—proximal tubule cells have an endocytic complex (apical canaliculi, vesicles, and vacuoles) actively involved in protein absorption.

—lateral borders of proximal tubule cells have extensive interdigitations that interlock them with one another.

—cells have extensive basal plasma membrane infoldings, which compartmentalize mitochondria.

—at least 80% of the sodium chloride and water, and all of the glucose, amino acids, and small proteins in the glomerular filtrate are absorbed in this part of the nephron.

—hydrogen ions are secreted in exchange for bicarbonate ions, and organic acids and bases are also secreted in this part of the nephron.

Descending Pars Recta (straight portion) of Proximal Tubule

—is also lined by a simple cuboidal epithelium having a prominent brush border.

—cells are shorter and less elaborate in shape than those of the proximal convoluted tubule, but they have the same general features.

—this region of the nephron is often damaged in acute renal failure and mercury poisoning.

—this segment constitutes the initial part (thick descending limb) of the loop of Henle.

Thin Limb of the Loop of Henle

—is composed of a descending limb, a loop, and an ascending limb, all of which are lined by a simple squamous epithelium.

—cells in this epithelium have nuclei that bulge into the lumen, and their surfaces possess only a few short microvilli.

—the thin limb has been separated into four distinct segments based on shape of cells, their content of organelles, the depth of their tight junctions, and their water permeability.

—is the region that forms the middle part of the loop of Henle.

Ascending Thick Limb (straight portion) of Distal Tubule

—is the third (and final) component of the loop of Henle.

—is lined by a simple cuboidal epithelium containing only a few microvilli.

—its nuclei occupy an apical position in the cells.

—mitochondria are compartmentalized within the interdigitations formed by the basal and lateral infoldings.

—cells transport ions from the lumen into the interstitium, and since this part of the nephron has a low permeability to water, the luminal fluid becomes hypotonic to the blood.

Macula Densa

—is a specific region of the distal tubule, lying near the afferent glomerular arteriole.

—is one component of the juxtaglomerular apparatus.

—cells are tall, narrow, and lined up closely together to form a row of nuclei that appear as a "dense spot" by light microscopy.

—cells are thought to monitor the fluid in the distal tubule and send a signal to the juxtaglomerular cells (modified smooth muscle cells) located in the afferent arteriole.

—signaling could occur via gap junctions present between these two cell types.

Distal Convoluted Tubule

—begins at the macula densa.

—is much shorter than the proximal convoluted tubule.

—cells have only a few luminal microvilli, and their nuclei occupy an apical position in the cytoplasm.

—extensive lateral interdigitations compartmentalize mitochondria in basal cytoplasmic infoldings.

—cells actively transport sodium ions from the filtrate into the interstitium.

Juxtaglomerular (JG) Apparatus

—is located at the vascular pole of the renal corpuscle.

—consists of four structures: modified smooth muscle cells of the afferent arteriole, of the efferent arteriole, the macula densa (of the distal tubule), and the extraglomerular mesangial cells.

Function of Juxtaglomerular Apparatus

—in response to a decrease in extracellular fluid volume (perhaps detected by the macula densa) the JG cells release renin (an enzyme).

Renin

—acts on angiotensinogen in the plasma, converting it to angiotensin I.

—in capillaries of the lung, angiotensin I is converted to angiotensin II, which causes release of aldosterone from the zona glomerulosa cells in the adrenal cortex.

Aldosterone

—stimulates distal tubule cells to retain sodium ions.

—water follows the sodium, and the fluid volume is increased in the extracellular compartment (thus correcting the initial problem).

Angiotensin II

—is also a potent vasoconstrictor, which acts to elevate the blood pressure.

Collecting Tubules

—have different functions, depending on their location in the kidney.

—in the cortex and medulla they respond to antidiurectic hormone (ADH), also known as vasopressin.

—in the medulla they play a primary role in producing a concentrated urine (by establishing a gradient due to the transport of urea from the tubular fluid into the renal interstitium).

Cortical Collecting Tubules

—are located primarily within the medullary ray, although a few arched collecting tubules exist within the cortical labyrinth.

—have two cell types, a light (principal) cell and a dark (intercalated) cell.

Light Cells

—are simple cuboidal in shape and have round centrally located nuclei.

—a single central cilium (flagellum) extends into the lumen from the surface of each light cell.

Dark Cells

—are fewer in number and have microplicae (folds) on their surface.

—apical cytoplasm of the dark cell contains many vesicles.

Medullary Collecting Tubule

—is similar in structure to the cortical collecting tubule.

—dark cells are present in outer medulla but absent in inner medulla.

—principal (light) cells increase in height, and in the inner medulla are the only cell type lining the collecting tubule.

Thick ascending segment
long. section

Thin segment
of Henle's loop
long. section

Collecting tubule

Blood vessels

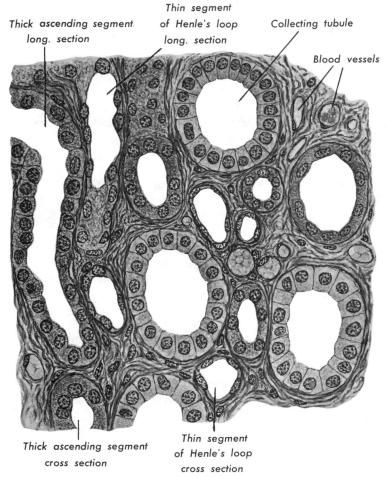

Thick ascending segment
cross section

Thin segment
of Henle's loop
cross section

Figure 16.4. Drawing of a section of the renal medulla. (From Kelly DE, Wood RL, Enders AC: *Bailey's Textbook of Microscopic Anatomy*, ed 18. Baltimore, Williams & Wilkins, 1984.)

Papillary Collecting Tubule (duct of Bellini)

—large collecting tubule formed from converging collecting tubules.
—consists only of principal cells and is a simple columnar epithelium.
—lumen of the duct of Bellini measures 200 to 300 μm in diameter.
—empties at the area cribrosa (a region having a sieve-like appearance) on the apex of a renal papilla.

Renal Interstitium

—is the connective tissue compartment in the kidney.
—in cortical interstitium are two main cell types: fibroblasts and mononuclear cells.
—in interstitium of the medulla, pericytes are present along the descending vasa recta.
—another cell type having long processes and containing many small lipid droplets (which probably contain a hormone that reduces blood pressure) is also common in medulla interstitium.

Blood Supply of Kidney
—is extensive (flow through both kidneys is about 1,200 ml/min).

Renal Artery
—and its branches enter the hilus, giving rise to interlobar arteries that travel between the renal pyramids.

Interlobar Arteries
—divide into several arcuate arteries that run along the corticomedullary junction, in a direction parallel with the surface of organ.
—small intralobular arteries arise from the arcuate arteries and enter the cortical tissue to pass between lobules.

Intralobular Arteries
—give rise to afferent (glomerular) arterioles, which supply the glomerular capillaries.

Efferent Glomerular Arterioles
—leave the glomerulus and give rise to an extensive peritubular capillary network that supplies the convoluted tubules.
—from glomeruli of juxtamedullary nephrons form thin-walled vessels called vasa recta, which are long straight capillaries that extend into the medullary pyramids.

Vasa Rectae
—form hairpin loops and ascend to form a countercurrent system of vessels called the vascular bundle (rete mirabile).
—these vessels drain into interlobular or arcuate veins, then into interlobar veins, which at the hilus form the renal vein.

Outermost Layers of Cortex
—are drained by superficial cortical veins, which join stellate veins and empty into interlobular and arcuate veins.

Deeper Regions of the Cortex
—are drained by deep cortical veins.

Excretory Passages

Components
—include the minor and major calyces, the renal pelvis, ureter, and urinary bladder.
—each of these passages has three layers, a mucosa (consisting of transitional epithelium lying on a subepithelial connective tissue), a muscularis, and an adventitia.

Ureter
—is the conduit between the renal pelvis and the urinary bladder.
—epithelium is thicker and has more cell layers than that in the calyces.
—upper two-thirds of ureter has an inner longitudinal and an outer circular layer of smooth muscle.
—lower one-third of ureter has an additional outer longitudinal layer of smooth muscle.
—contraction of these muscle layers produces peristaltic waves, which propel the urine along so that it enters the bladder in spurts.

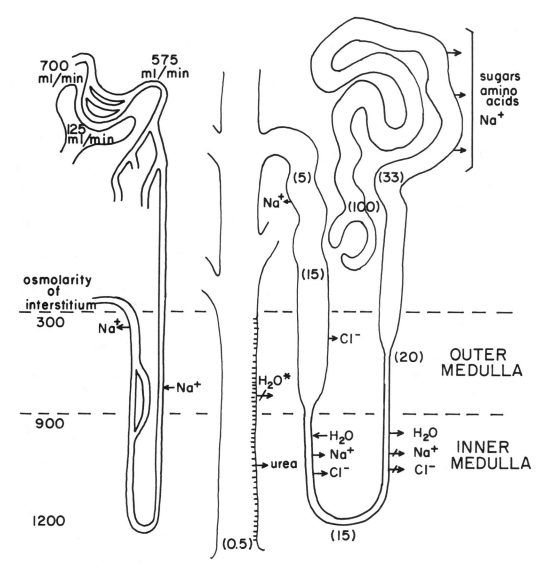

Figure 16.5. Diagram of the histophysiologic relationship between the uriniferous tubule and the renal interstitium. (From Kelly DE, Wood RL, Enders AC: *Bailey's Textbook of Microscopic Anatomy*, ed 18. Baltimore, Williams & Wilkins, 1984.)

Urinary Bladder

—is lined by a layer of transitional epithelium several cell layers thick.

—lumen of the bladder has a scalloped contour in the relaxed state, due to the dome-shaped surface cells.

—lining cells have a thick asymmetrical plasmalemma, which displays a unique substructure (when viewed in the transmission electron microscope after freeze fracture).

—plaques in the form of hexagonally arranged subunits are observed, but their functional significance remains obscure.

—cytoplasm of the surface cell has flattened elliptical vesicles, which insert themselves into the plasma membrane (to rapidly expand the area when the bladder is stretched).

—epithelium has a remarkable ability to change its morphology in the relaxed versus the distended state.

—a thin basal lamina underlies the transitional epithelium, and beneath it is fibroelastic connective tissue.

—muscularis of the bladder is thick and consists of smooth muscle arranged in an inner longitudinal, middle circular, and outer longitudinal layer.

Male Urethra

—conveys urine from the urinary bladder to the outside.

—also serves as a passageway for semen during ejaculation.

—is divided into prostatic, membranous, and cavernous portions.

—transitional epithelium lines the prostatic portion, while pseudostratified or stratified columnar epithelium lines the remaining portions.

—beneath a thin basement membrane is the subepithelial connective tissue, where mucus-secreting glands (of Littrè) may be found.

—muscularis has an inner longitudinal and an outer circular layer.

—at distal end of the cavernous urethra is the fossa navicularis, lined by stratified squamous epithelium.

Female Urethra

—is a short passageway from the urinary bladder to the outside.

—is lined primarily by stratified squamous epithelium, but has patches of pseudostratified columnar epithelium.

—mucus-secreting glands (of Littrè) are located in the subepithelial connective tissue.

—muscularis is composed of an inner longitudinal and an outer circular layer of smooth muscle.

REVIEW TESTS

URINARY SYSTEM

16.1. A medullary ray
1. contains arched collecting tubules
2. contains thick ascending limbs of the loop of Henle
3. does not extend into the cortex
4. lies at the center of a renal lobule

16.2. A nephron includes which of the following?
1. a renal corpuscle
2. a distal convoluted tubule
3. a thin limb of the loop of Henle
4. a collecting tubule

16.3. Podocytes
1. are classified as modified simple squamous epithelial cells
2. line the parietal layer of Bowman's capsule
3. have tiny extensions called pedicels
4. phagocytose large protein molecules in the ultrafiltrate

16.4. The juxtaglomerular apparatus
1. is located at the vascular pole of the renal corpuscle
2. includes the mesangial cells of the glomerular tuft
3. produces renin
4. functions to cause a decrease in blood pressure

16.5. The cortical collecting tubules
1. include the large ducts of Bellini
2. are lined by two cell types
3. empty into the area cribrosa
4. respond to the hormone vasopressin

16.6. The urethra in males
1. serves as a passage for semen
2. is lined exclusively by transitional epithelium
3. has a muscularis formed by an inner longitudinal and outer circular layer of smooth muscle
4. lacks a well-defined muscularis

DIRECTIONS: Select the *one* lettered structure on the electron micrograph (Fig. 16.6) that *best* corresponds to the numbered word, phrase, or description listed below. Each letter may be used once, more than once, or not at all.

16.7. pedicel

16.8. Bowman's (capsular) space

16.9. endothelium

16.10. the major barrier for the selective filtration of proteins

16.11. the basal lamina

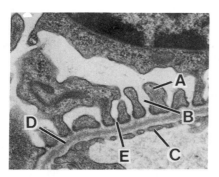

Figure 16.6. From Gartner LP, Hiatt JL: *Atlas of Histology*. Baltimore, Williams & Wilkins, 1987.

ANSWERS AND EXPLANATIONS

URINARY SYSTEM

16.1. C (2 and 4)

A medullary ray is formed by the straight portions of tubules projecting from the medulla into the cortex and giving the appearance of striations or rays. A renal lobule, by definition, consists of a centrally located medullary ray together with its closely associated cortical tissue.

16.2. A (1, 2, and 3)

A nephron includes a renal corpuscle, a proximal tubule (convoluted and straight portions), the thin limb of the loop of Henle, the ascending thick limb of Henle's loop, macula densa, and the distal convoluted tubule. All of these structures originated embryonically from the metanephrogenic blastema. The collecting tubule, which originated from the ureteric bud, is not considered to be part of the nephron.

16.3. B (1 and 3)

Podocytes form the visceral (not parietal) layer within Bowman's capsule and constitute a modified simple squamous epithelium. These cells have primary processes that give rise to smaller secondary processes (pedicels), which are separated from one another by filtration slits (bridged by diaphragms of filamentous material). Podocytes are not phagocytic cells, and protein molecules having a molecular weight greater than 69,000 are not normally present in the ultrafiltrate.

16.4. B (1 and 3)

The juxtaglomerular apparatus is located at the vascular pole of the renal corpuscle. It includes four structures: the afferent arteriole, which contains the juxtaglomerular cells and their renin granules; the macula densa of the distal tubule; the extraglomerular mesangial cells (lacis cells; Polkissen cells); and the efferent arteriole. The function of the juxtaglomerular apparatus is to trigger mechanisms that result in an increase in blood pressure.

16.5. C (2 and 4)

The cortical collecting tubules are characterized by two cell types: a principal (light) cell and a dark (intercalated) cell. These tubules respond to vasopressin (ADH) by removing water from their lumens and producing a more concentrated urine. The large ducts of Bellini are present only in the papilla and empty their contents into the minor calyces by way of the area cribrosa.

16.6. B (1 and 3)

In males the urethra serves not only as a conduit for conveying urine from the bladder to the outside but also as a passageway for semen (during ejaculation). It is divided into three separate segments, each of which is lined by a different type of epithelium. Its muscularis is well defined and consists of an inner longitudinal and outer circular layer of smooth muscle.

For questions **16.7** to **16.11**, refer to Figure 16.6.

16.7. A

16.8. B

16.9. C

16.10. D

16.11. D

256

17

Female Reproductive System

Female Reproductive System

—consists of the ovaries, oviducts, uterus, vagina, and external genitalia. The mammary glands will also be discussed in this chapter.

—functions in the propagation of the species and is controlled by a complex interplay of psychological, neural, and humoral factors.

External Genitalia and the Breasts

—undergo marked changes in females at the onset of puberty (about age 13), which is marked by menarche, the first menstrual event.

Menstrual Cycles

—continue monthly until the end of the female's reproductive period, which culminates in menopause, the cessation of menstruation.

Ovary

—is a small, almond-shaped body, located retroperitoneally and attached to the posterior body wall by the broad ligament, via the mesovarium.

—its capsule is invested by a modification of the peritoneum, the germinal epithelium, a simple squamous (or cuboidal) epithelium

—is subdivided into the cortex, containing ovarian follicles (at various stages of development), and a vascular medulla.

Cortex

Tunica Albuginea

—is the dense irregular collagenous connective tissue capsule of the ovary.

Primordial Follicles

—are composed of a primary oocyte (arrested in the first meiotic division) and a single layer of squamous follicular cells.

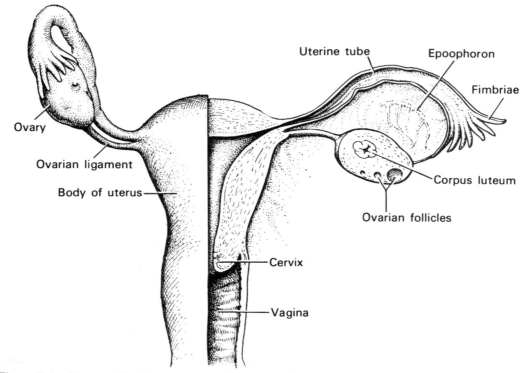

Figure 17.1. Diagram of the female reproductive system. (From Copenhaver WM, Kelly DE, Wood RL: *Bailey's Textbook of Histology*, ed 17. Baltimore, Williams & Wilkins, 1978.)

Follicular Cells
—are separated by a basal lamina from the surrounding stroma (the highly cellular connective tissue of the ovary).
—are attached to each other by desmosomes.

Oocyte
—displays a prominent, acentric, vesicular appearing nucleus, possessing a single nucleolus.
—its cytoplasm contains many Golgi bodies, mitochondria, profiles of rough endoplasmic reticulum, and well-developed annulate lamellae.

Primary Follicles (unilaminar)
—are similar to primordial follicles, except that the follicular cells are somewhat larger and are cuboidal in shape.

Primary Follicles (multilaminar)
—are composed of several layers of follicular cells, now referred to as granulosa cells, which communicate with each other via gap junctions.

Granulosa Cells
—are separated from the primary oocyte by an amorphous layer of glycoprotein, the zona pellucida.

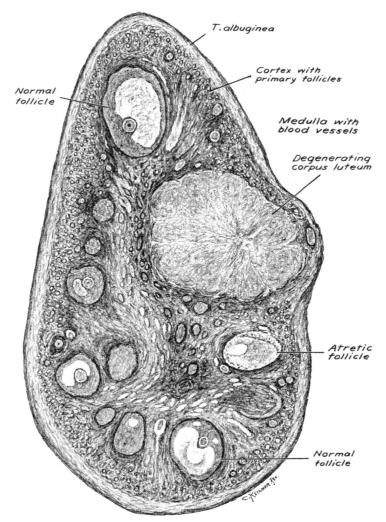

Figure 17.2. Drawing of a section of the ovary. (From Copenhaver WM, Kelly DE, Wood RL: *Bailey's Textbook of Histology*, ed 17. Baltimore, Williams & Wilkins, 1978.)

Microvilli

—from the oocyte and narrow processes from the granulosa cells extend into and contact each other within the substance of the zona pellucida.

Membrana Limitans Externa

—is the thickened basal lamina that separates the granulosa cells from the stroma.

Stroma

—begins to circumscribe the follicle, forming the two layers, the cellular theca interna and the fibrous theca externa.

Secondary Follicle (antral follicle)

—is larger than the primary follicle.

Liquor Folliculi

—an accumulation of a fluid in the intercellular spaces of the granulosa cells distinguishes the secondary from the multilaminar primary follicle.

Oocyte

—is acentrically positioned and has reached its final size (about 150 μm diameter).

Call-Exner Bodies

—are dense spherical structures that are also present in the intercellular spaces.

Graafian (mature) Follicle

—is approximately 2.5 cm in diameter.

—is evident as a large bulge on the surface of the ovary and represents the final stage of follicular development, just prior to ovulation.

Liquor Folliculi

—has coalesced to form a region of fluid contained in a space, called the antrum.

Antrum

—is surrounded by several layers of granulosa cells (the membrana granulosa).

Cumulus Oophorus

—is a peninsula-like structure, composed of granulosa cells, that juts into the antrum.

Granulosa Cells

—surround the zona pellucida and the primary oocyte.

Oocyte

—is separated from the granulosa cells by the thickened zona pellucida.

Microvilli

—of the oocyte and processes of the granulosa cells immediately adjacent to the oocyte (cells that form the corona radiata) contact each other via gap junctions and also form gap junctions with the oocyte.

Membrana Limitans Externa

—separates the granulosa cells from the cellular theca interna.

Theca Interna

—manufactures the precursor of the female sex hormone.

Theca Externa

—is collagenous and contains many blood vessels that provide nourishment to the theca interna.

Ovulation

—is the release of the oocyte (with its attendant cumulus cells) from the graafian follicle and the ovary.

Primary Oocyte

—completes its first meiotic division just prior to ovulation, forming the secondary oocyte and the first polar body, and begins the second meiotic division.

Secondary Oocyte

—and its attendant cumulus cells (the corona radiata) leave the follicle via a small gap.

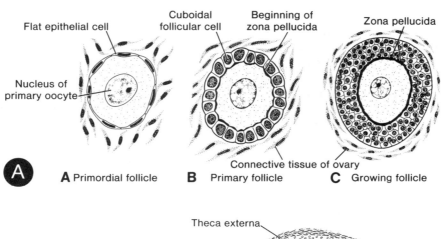

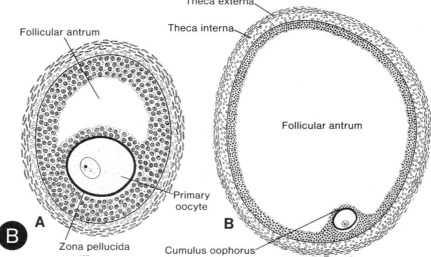

Figure 17.3. **A**: diagram of various stages of follicular development. **A**, primordial follicles; **B**, unilaminar primary follicle; **C**, multilaminar primary follicle. (From Sadler TW: *Langman's Medical Embryology*, ed 5. Baltimore, Williams & Wilkins, 1985.) **B**: diagram of a secondary follicle (**A**) and a graafian follicle (**B**). (From Sadler TW: *Langman's Medical Embryology*, ed 5. Baltimore, Williams & Wilkins, 1985.)

—gaps are formed in the compressed capsule, germinal epithelium, and wall of the graafian follicle (the region of the stigma on the ovarian surface).

Corpus Hemorrhagicum

—is the hemorrhaged remainder of the folded and modified follicular structure.

—is subsequently transformed into the corpus luteum.

Membrana Limitans Externa

—separating the theca interna and the membrana granulosa disappears.

Secondary Oocyte

—with its corona radiata enters (after ovulation) the fimbriated end (infundibulum) of the oviduct.

Fertilization

—usually takes place within the ampulla of the oviduct.

—occurs when the spermatozoon penetrates the corona radiata, zona pellucida, and the plasmalemma of the secondary oocyte.

—triggers the resumption and completion of the second meiotic division, with the subsequent formation of the ovum and the second polar body.

—male pronucleus (from the spermatozoon) and the female pronucleus (from the ovum) then fuse, forming a diploid (2N) cell, known as a zygote.

Corpus Luteum

—is composed of two major cell types: the granulosa lutein cells (modified granulosa cells) and the theca lutein cells (modified theca interna cells).

—has many capillaries.

Granulosa Lutein Cells

—are large (30 μm diameter).

—are pale cells with abundant rough and smooth endoplasmic reticulum, numerous mitochondria, a well-developed Golgi apparatus, and many lipid droplets.

Theca Lutein Cells

—are smaller (15 μm diameter), more darkly stained, display a varied organelle population and have numerous lipid droplets.

In the Absence of Pregnancy

—the corpus luteum becomes nonfunctional within two weeks (the corpus luteum of menstruation).

In the Event of Pregnancy

—the corpus luteum retains its full functional capacity for about half a year, and then its activity decreases until term (the corpus luteum of pregnancy).

Corpus Albicans

—is formed after the corpus luteum ceases to function.

Corpus Luteum

—degenerates, its cells undergo autolysis (and its remnants are phagocytosed by macrophages).

—becomes invaded by fibroblasts, becomes fibrotic, and shrinks until it is evident merely as a small scar on the surface of the ovary.

Atretic Follicles

—are follicles in various stages of maturation that are undergoing active degeneration.

—are commonly present in the ovary, since during the menstrual cycle after one follicle releases its oocyte, the remaining developing follicles undergo degeneration.

—are characterized by

  —pyknotic changes in the nucleus of the oocyte
  —dissolution of the zona pellucida
  —dispersal and degeneration of the follicular (granulosa) cells
  —hyalinization of the basal lamina (which becomes known as the glassy membrane)

Interstitial Cells

—are scarce in the ovary of the human female but are thought to be derived from the theca interna. They produce androgens.

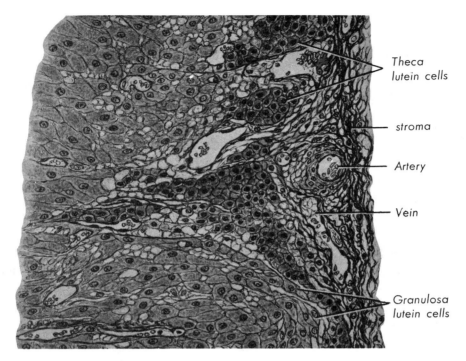

Theca lutein cells

stroma

Artery

Vein

Granulosa lutein cells

Figure 17.4. Drawing of a section of the corpus luteum. (From Copenhaver WM, Kelly DE, Wood RL: *Bailey's Textbook of Histology*, ed 17. Baltimore, Williams & Wilkins, 1978.)

Medulla
—of the ovary contains large blood vessels that provide blood supply to the cortex.

Blood Vessels
—enter and leave the medulla at the hilus, where large epithelioid (hilus) cells form clumps in their vicinity.

Hilus Cells
—are similar in structure to the interstitial cells of Leydig (in the testes) and probably produce androgens.

Stroma
—also contains loose connective tissue rich in elastic and collagen fibers, housing numerous fibroblasts.

Histophysiology of the Ovary

Gonadotropin-Releasing Hormone (GnRH)
—from the hypothalamus causes the release of follicle-stimulating (FSH) and luteinizing hormones (LH) by the pars anterior of the pituitary gland.

FSH
—stimulates the growth and development of the ovarian follicles resulting in:
  —theca interna cells manufacture androgens, which the granulosa cells convert into estrogens and release.
  —granulosa cells also secrete folliculostatin.

—estrogen and folliculostatin blood levels become sufficiently high by approximately the 14th day of the menstrual cycle to inhibit the release of FSH and facilitate an increase in LH secretion.

LH

—surge triggers the transformation of the primary oocyte into a secondary oocyte and promotes its ovulation from a graafian follicle.

  —follicle that released its oocyte is subsequently transformed into a corpus luteum that produces estrogen and progesterone.

Estrogen

—continues to inhibit FSH release (by suppressing the release of GnRH).

Progesterone

—inhibits the release of LH (by suppressing the release of GnRH) but promotes development of the uterine endometrium.

In the Event of Pregnancy

—the syncytiotrophoblasts of the developing placenta will manufacture chorionic gonadotropins.
—chorionic gonadotropin maintains the corpus luteum of pregnancy.

In the Absence of Pregnancy

—neither LH nor chorionic gonadotropins are present and the corpus luteum begins to atrophy.
—lack of estrogen and progesterone also permits the pituitary to release FSH and LH, thus re-initiating the ovarian cycle.

Oviduct

Oviduct (fallopian tube)

—is a muscular tube (12 cm long) that functions to convey the zygote to the uterus.
—is the most frequent site of fertilization.
—is subdivided into four regions: the infundibulum (with its fimbriated end); the ampulla (the usual site of fertilization); the isthmus; and the pars interstitialis (intramural portion), which traverses the wall of the uterus.
—its wall consists of three main layers: the mucosa, muscularis, and the serosa.

Figure 17.5. Drawing of a cross section of the infundibulum of the oviduct. (From Copenhaver WM, Kelly DE, Wood RL: *Bailey's Textbook of Histology*, ed 17. Baltimore, Williams & Wilkins, 1978.)

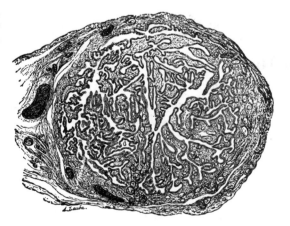

Mucosa

—of the oviduct is extensively folded (in a longitudinal direction) in the infundibulum.
—degree of folding progressively decreases in the remaining three segments.

Epithelium

—is simple columnar and consists of two types of cells: peg cells and ciliated cells.

Peg Cells

—secrete a nutrient-rich medium that nourishes the spermatozoa and zygote.
—cytoplasm is rich in rough endoplasmic reticulum, displays a well-developed Golgi apparatus, and contains many apically located electron-dense secretory granules.

Ciliated Cells

—possess many cilia, which beat toward the lumen of the uterus.
—may facilitate the transport of the developing embryo to the uterus, but muscular contraction could be equally important.

Lamina Propria

—of the oviduct consists of loose connective tissue containing reticular fibers, fibroblasts, mast cells, and lymphoid cells.
—is interposed between the epithelium and the muscularis.

Muscularis

—is composed of an ill-defined inner circular and outer longitudinal layer of smooth muscle.
—its contraction is thought to play a role in moving the ovum toward the uterus.

Serosa

—is a connective tissue layer lined by a simple squamous epithelium that envelops the muscularis.
—contains blood vessels, lymphatics, and nerves.
—its simple squamous epithelium represents the peritoneal lining.

Uterus

—a pear-shaped organ, is subdivided into three regions: the fundus, body (corpus), and cervix.
—houses the developing embryo and fetus during pregnancy.
—endometrium of this organ participates in the formation of the placenta (which provides nourishment for the developing fetus).
—as the fetus enlarges, the uterus increases in size and acquires a thick muscular coat, the myometrium.
—myometrium contracts at parturition, assisting the expulsion of the fetus and the placenta.
—wall of the uterus consists of the endometrium, myometrium, and the adventitia (or serosa).

Endometrium

—undergoes hormonally modulated cyclic alterations, known as the menstrual cycle.
—is subdivided into two layers, the thick superficial functional layer and the deeper basal layer. The separation between the two layers is indistinct.

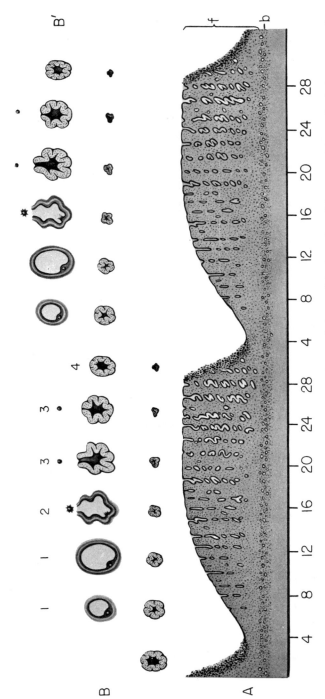

Figure 17.6. Diagram illustrating the relationship between menstruation, ovulation, and the formation of the corpus luteum. **A**, uterine mucosa; **b**, basal layer; **f**, functional layer; **B**, ovarian cycle; **1**, maturing follicle; **2**, ovulation; **3**, corpus luteum; **4** and remaining figures, degeneration of the corpus luteum; numbers at base (4 to 28), indicate days of the menstrual cycle. (From Copenhaver WM, Kelly DE, Wood RL: *Bailey's Textbook of Histology*, ed 17. Baltimore, Williams & Wilkins, 1978.)

127

Epithelium

—lining the surface is simple columnar, consisting of two types of cells, secretory and ciliated.

Glands

—are composed of similar types of cells, but they contain fewer ciliated cells.

Stroma

—is almost like mesenchymal connective tissue (with an abundance of reticular fibers and stellate-shaped cells). Macrophages and lymphoid elements are also present.

—functional layer (functionalis) is the thick superficial layer of the endometrium that is sloughed and reestablished monthly due to cyclic hormonal changes.

—basal layer (basalis) is the thin deeper layer of the endometrium that is preserved during menstruation.

Endometrial Glands

—extend through the basal layer.

—after the functional layer is sloughed, cells for reepithelialization of the endometrium are derived from the base of these glands.

Vascular Supply

—of the endometrium is derived from the arcuate arteries located in the stratum vasculare of the myometrium. Two types of arteries arise from here: helical and straight.

Helical Arteries

—extend into the functional layer.

Straight Arteries

—terminate in the basal layer.

Menstrual Cycle

—has three phases: follicular (proliferative), luteal (secretory), and menstrual.

Follicular (proliferative) Phase

—follows the menstrual phase when the functional layer has been sloughed and the luminal surface is in the process of being reepithelialized (from cells in the base of the uterine glands).

—proliferation of the glandular, connective tissue, and vascular elements (helical arteries) occurs concurrently.

—lamina propria becomes reestablished, as the functional layer is renewed.

—stromal cells undergo the decidual reaction, in that they amass glycogen, enlarge, and become pale-staining decidual cells.

—near the end of the proliferative phase (day 15) the glands become coiled and their cells begin to store glycogen.

—helical arteries extend approximately two-thirds of the way into the endometrium.

Luteal (secretory) Phase

—begins shortly after ovulation and is characterized by a thickening of the endo-metrium, from edema and the secretion by the endometrial glands.

—glands become coiled, their lumina contain secretory products, and, temporarily, the nuclei of their cells become apically oriented (due to the basal accumulation of glycogen).

—helical arteries become longer and more coiled, so that they reach the superficial aspect of the functional layer.

Menstrual Phase

—begins approximately two weeks after ovulation in the absence of pregnancy.

—absence of progesterone causes long-term vasoconstriction of the helical arteries, which results in ischemia and subsequent necrosis of the functional layer.

—sudden, intermittent vasodilation of the helical arteries is responsible for dislodging the necrotic tissue.

—necrotic tissue enters the uterine lumen to become menstrual discharge.

—basal layer is not sloughed and does not become necrotic, since it is supplied by short straight vessels that do not undergo prolonged vasoconstriction.

Myometrium

—is the thick smooth muscle coat of the uterus.

—is composed of three poorly delineated layers: inner and outer longitudinal and a thick middle circular layer.

—circular layer is richly vascularized and is often referred to as the stratum vasculare.

—during pregnancy the myometrium thickens due to the hypertrophy of individual smooth muscle cells, an increase in the number of muscle fibers, and increase in connective tissue components.

—activity of the myometrium decreases until parturition (probably due to the hormone relaxin produced by the corpus luteum).

—at parturition the hormone oxytocin (released by the neurohypophysis) assists in triggering the myometrium to undergo powerful contractions.

Cervix

—is the region of the uterus that projects into the vagina.

—its wall is composed of dense collagenous connective tissue interspersed with numerous elastic fibers and a few smooth muscle cells.

—its epithelium is a simple columnar (mucus-secreting) epithelium except for the inferior portion that is continuous with the lining of the vagina and is covered by a stratified squamous nonkeratinized epithelium.

—branched cervical glands secrete a serous fluid around the time of ovulation that facilitates the entry of spermatozoa into the uterine lumen.

—during pregnancy these glands produce a thick, viscous secretion that hinders the entry of spermatozoa (and microorganisms) into the uterine cavity.

—prior to parturition the cervix becomes dilated and softens due to the lysis of collagen in response to the hormone relaxin.

Serosa (or adventitia)

—covers the myometrium.

Implantation

Zygote

—via mitotic activity, is transformed into a multicellular structure.

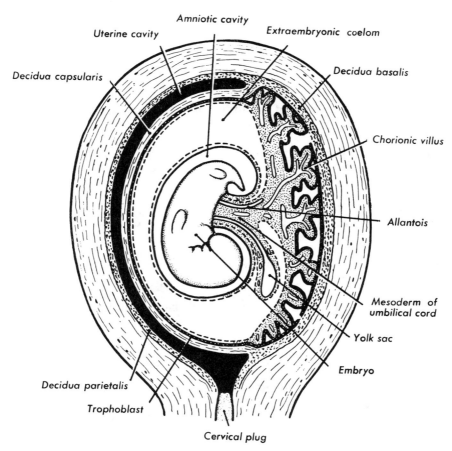

Figure 17.7. Diagram of the fetal and decidual membranes. (From Copenhaver WM, Kelly DE, Wood RL: *Bailey's Textbook of Histology*, ed 17. Baltimore, Williams & Wilkins, 1978.)

Trophoblasts

—invade the endometrium and facilitate the implantation of the embryo.

—give rise to two layers, the cytotrophoblasts and the syncytiotrophoblasts.

Syncytiotrophoblasts

—secrete three hormones: estrogens, chorionic gonadotropin, and placental lactogen.

—form lacunae (extracellular cavities), which receive blood from the arterial supply of the mother and are drained by maternal veins.

Primary Villi

—are finger-like projections of the syncytiotrophoblasts (with a core of cytotrophoblasts) that protrude into the lacunae.

Decidua

—is the name given to the endometrium subsequent to implantation.

—is subdivided into three regions, with respect to the developing embyro: decidua basalis, capsularis, and parietalis.

Decidua Basalis
—is located between the myometrium and the embryo.

Decidua Capsularis
—is located between the uterine lumen and the embryo.

Decidua Parietalis
—is located between the lumen of the uterus and the myometrium.

Chorion
—is formed by the trophoblasts, in conjunction with the extraembryonic mesenchyme.
—completely surrounds the developing embryo and has two regions: the chorion laeve and chorion frondosum.

Chorion Laeve
—smoother and less developed, is found at the decidua capsularis.

Chorion Frondosum
—highly developed, is located at the decidua basalis.

Secondary Villi
—are formed when the cores of the primary villi become invaded by extraembryonic mesenchyme.

Placenta
—is a transient structure, consisting of a maternal portion (arising from the decidua basalis) and a fetal portion (arising from the chorion).
—permits the exchange of various materials between the maternal and fetal circulatory systems.
—exchange occurs without mixing of the two blood supplies.
—forms progesterone, human chorionic gonadotropin, and human chorionic somatomammotropin (a lactogenic and growth-promoting hormone).
—produces estrogen, with the assistance of the liver and adrenal cortex of the fetus.

Fetal Portion
—consists of the chorionic plate from which arise the secondary villi.
—during the first half of pregnancy, large, vacuolated macrophages (Hofbauer cells) are present in the connective tissue of secondary villi.
—connective tissue (extraembryonic mesenchyme): cores of the secondary villi become invaded by capillaries, thus transforming them into chorionic (tertiary) villi.
—during the second half of the pregnancy, cytotrophoblast and syncytiotrophoblast cells merge.
—merging reduces the thickness of the barrier between the maternal blood in the intervillous spaces (formed from the expanded and coalesced lacunae) and the fetal blood in capillaries of the chorionic villi.
—nuclei of the syncytiotrophoblasts congregate to form syncytial knots.

Villi
—may either be attached to the decidua basalis (anchoring villi) or free floating and blindly ending in the intervillous space (terminal villi).
—are mostly terminal villi.

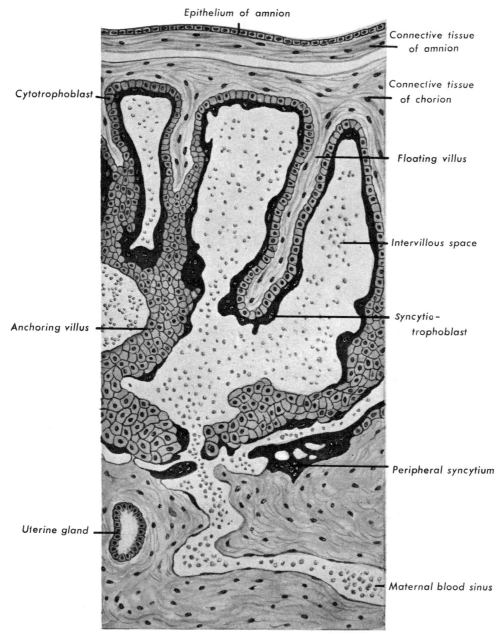

Figure 17.8. Schematic drawing of the placenta. (From Copenhaver WM, Kelly DE, Wood RL: *Bailey's Textbook of Histology*, ed 17. Baltimore, Williams & Wilkins, 1978.)

Maternal Portion

—consists of the decidua basalis, which provides an arterial supply and venous drainage for the lacunae.

—tertiary villi are enveloped by maternal blood.

—during the first half of pregnancy, some of the connective tissue cells of the decidua basalis transform into decidual cells that manufacture prolactin.

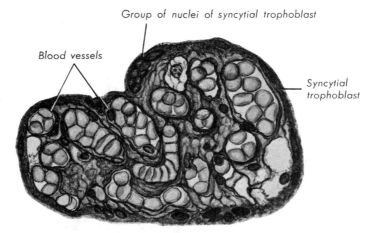

Figure 17.9. Drawing of a cross section of a secondary placental villus. (From Copenhaver WM, Kelly DE, Wood RL: *Bailey's Textbook of Histology*, ed 17. Baltimore, Williams & Wilkins, 1978.)

Vagina

—a fibromuscular tube whose wall is composed of three layers: an inner mucosa (whose deep layer is a submucosa), a middle muscularis, and an external adventitia.

Mucosa

—is lined by a thick, stratified squamous nonkeratinized epithelium, although some of the cells of the superficial layers may contain keratohyalin granules.

Epithelial Cells

—also contain glycogen, which is used by the vaginal bacterial flora to produce lactic acid, which lowers the pH during the follicular phase of the menstrual cycle.

Lamina Propria

—is composed of a fibroelastic connective tissue, rich in elastic fibers and lymphoid elements.

—its deep portion propria is highly vascular, and some consider it analogous to a submucosa.

—glands are not present in the wall of the vagina.

Muscularis

—is composed of a thin inner circular and a thicker outer longitudinal layer of smooth muscle. The external orifice of the vagina is circumscribed by skeletal muscle fibers.

Adventitia

—is composed of fibroelastic connective tissue that fixes the vagina to the surrounding structures. Blood vessels and nerves are present in this layer.

External Genitalia (Vulva)

—is richly innervated.

—includes the labia majora, labia minora, clitoris, and the mucus-secreting vestibular glands.

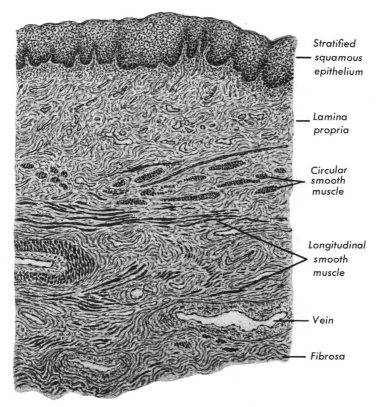

Figure 17.10. Drawing of a longitudinal section of the vagina. (From Copenhaver WM, Kelly DE, Wood RL: *Bailey's Textbook of Histology*, ed 17. Baltimore, Williams & Wilkins, 1978.)

Labia Majora

—are fat-laden folds of skin (corresponding to the scrotum), whose inner aspects are devoid of hair, whereas their outer aspects possess hair.

—both surfaces contain sebaceous glands and sweat glands.

—have a thin layer of smooth muscle (corresponding to the dartos muscle) in their wall.

Labia Minora

—are folds of skin that possess a core of highly vascular, spongy connective tissue containing elastic fibers.

—hair follicles are absent, but sebaceous and sweat glands are numerous.

Vestibule

—is the space partially enclosed by the two labia minora.

—is partially occluded by a thin membrane, the hymen, in a virgin.

Clitoris

—is composed of two small, cylindrical erectile bodies (homologue of the dorsal aspect of the penis), which terminate in the prepuce-covered glans clitoridis.

—stroma of the clitoris is rich in blood vessels and contains many sensory nerve fibers and specialized nerve endings, such as Meissner's and Pacinian corpuscles.

Vestibular Glands

—are of two types: glands of Bartholin and the minor vestibular glands.

Glands of Bartholin

—are large and two in number.
—open into the vestibule on the inner surface of the labia minora.
—resemble the male bulbourethral glands.

Minor Vestibular Glands

—are numerous and small.
—are located around the clitoris and the urethra.
—resemble the glands of Littrè.
—produce a mucous secretion.

Mammary Gland

—produces milk, a lipid- and protein-rich fluid that nourishes the newborn.
—secretes, for the first few days after birth, colostrum, a fluid rich in cells, lipid, and antibodies (mainly secretory IgA).
—immunoglobulins provide an immunological defense for the neonate.
—is composed of about two dozen compound tubuloalveolar glands, each of which has its own lactiferous sinus and duct that opens at the apex of the nipple.
—male and female mammary glands are identical until puberty.
—at puberty, mammary glands in the female acquire adipose tissue in their stroma, thus increasing their size due to hormonal changes.
—terminal ductules are formed in the female mammary gland at puberty.
—alveoli form only during pregnancy by additional growth from the terminal ductules.
—when secreting milk (during lactation), mammary gland is said to be "active."
—is said to be "resting" at all other times.

Milk

—is released from the mammary gland via the milk ejection reflex, in response to external stimuli related to suckling by the baby.
—reflex involves release of oxytocin (by the pars nervosa of the pituitary gland), which induces contraction in myoepithelial cells located around the alveoli and ducts.
—is forced into the larger ducts and out of the gland.

Resting Gland

—is composed of lactiferous sinuses and lactiferous ducts and their branches.

Lactiferous Sinuses

—are lined by stratified squamous epithelium near their opening on the nipple and by a stratified cuboidal epithelium along the remainder of their length.

Lactiferous Ducts

—are lined by a stratified cuboidal epithelium containing the normal complement of organelles and adhering to one another by desmosomes and zonulae occludentes.

Myoepithelial Cells

—underlie lactiferous ducts in most areas.
—are analogous to smooth muscle fibers.

Basal Lamina
—separates the epithelial components from the stroma.

Active Gland
—is much larger than that in the resting phase. This increase in size is due to the proliferation of the terminal ductules to form alveoli.

Alveoli
—are composed of alveolar cells, which secrete lipid, casein, and lactose.

Alveolar Cells
—are surrounded by an incomplete layer of myoepithelial cells.
—are richly endowed with rough endoplasmic reticulum, several Golgi regions, numerous mitochondria, and many vesicles.
—possess abundant lipid droplets and milk protein (casein).
—during lactation the number of casein droplets and lipid in the alveoli increases and the secretory cells become low cuboidal.

Mode of Secretion
—lipid secretion appears to be apocrine (a portion of the cytoplasm might be released with the lipid).
—proteins are delivered into the lumen via the merocrine (exocytosis) method.

Nipple
—is a skin-covered conical protuberance composed of dense collagenous connective tissue interlaced with smooth muscle fibers.
—contains the openings of the lactiferous ducts.

Areola
—is a circular region of pigmented skin surrounding the nipple.
—becomes more deeply pigmented during pregnancy and contains the areolar glands (of Montgomery).

REVIEW TESTS

FEMALE REPRODUCTIVE SYSTEM

DIRECTIONS: *One* or *more* of the given completions is/are correct. Choose answer:
- A. if only **1**, **2**, and **3** are correct
- B. if only **1** and **3** are correct
- C. if only **2** and **4** are correct
- D. if only **4** is correct
- E. if **all** are correct

17.1. The capsule of the ovary
1. is composed of dense irregular collagenous connective tissue
2. is composed of dense elastic connective tissue
3. is covered by a germinal epithelium
4. possesses an inner layer, known as the tunica vasculosa

17.2. The primordial follicle
1. has flattened follicular cells
2. contains a primary oocyte
3. possesses no Call-Exner bodies
4. has a thick zona pellucida

17.3. The corpus luteum
1. produces LH
2. produces FSH
3. derives its parenchymal cells from the theca externa
4. becomes the corpus albicans

17.4. Luteinizing hormone
1. is responsible for the completion of the second meiotic division
2. triggers ovulation
3. suppresses the release of estrogens
4. induces the completion of the first meiotic division

17.5. The epithelium of the oviduct
1. is composed of a simple columnar epithelium
2. has peg cells
3. has ciliated cells
4. functions in nourishing spermatozoa

17.6. The basal layer of the uterine endometrium
1. becomes sloughed off
2. has no glands
3. is supplied by helical arteries
4. is supplied by straight arteries

17.7. The uterine endometrium undergoes the following phases:
1. luteal
2. active
3. follicular
4. resting

17.8. Primary villi of the chorion possess
1. blood vessels
2. cytotrophoblasts
3. extraembryonic mesenchyme
4. syncytiotrophoblasts

DIRECTIONS: Each of the following questions contains five suggested answers. Choose the *one* that is *best* in each case.

17.9. The fetal portion of the placenta

A. contains maternal blood
B. possesses Hofbauer cells
C. consists of the chorionic plate
D. consists of the decidua basalis
E. produces the hormone prolactin

17.10. The mucosa of the vagina

A. is lined by stratified columnar epithelium
B. is lined by stratified squamous keratinized epithelium
C. possesses no elastic fibers
D. secretes glycogen
E. secretes lactic acid

17.11. *One* of the following statements is not true concerning the mammary gland:

A. contains lactiferous ducts
B. produces colostrum
C. is identical in males and females prior to puberty
D. contains myoepithelial cells
E. forms alveoli only during menstruation

DIRECTIONS: The following questions or statements refer to the photomicrograph (Fig. 17.11). The letters on the figure are answers to the numbered items appearing below the photomicrograph. For each numbered item select the *one* letter that *best* corresponds to that item. Each letter may be used once, more than once, or not at all.

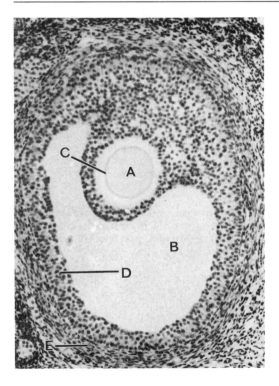

Figure 17.11. From Gartner LP, Hiatt JL: *Atlas of Histology*. Baltimore, Williams & Wilkins, 1987.)

17.12. theca interna

17.13. liquor folliculi

17.14. membrana granulosa

17.15. antrum

ANSWERS AND EXPLANATIONS

FEMALE REPRODUCTIVE SYSTEM

17.1. B (1 and 3)
The ovarian capsule is composed of dense irregular collagenous connective tissue, covered by the germinal epithelium, which is part of the peritoneum.

17.2. A (1, 2, and 3)
The primordial follicle is composed of a flattened layer of follicular cells surrounding the primary oocyte. Call-Exner bodies and the thick zona pellucida are found in latter stages of follicular development.

17.3. D (4)
LH and FSH are hormones produced by the pituitary gland. Parenchymal cells of the corpus luteum are derived from the theca interna and the membrana granulosa. The corpus albicans is formed after the corpus luteum ceases to function.

17.4. C (2 and 4)
The sudden surge of LH is responsible for triggering the completion of the first meiotic division as well as for inducing ovulation. This hormone does not affect the second meiotic division nor does it suppress estrogen production.

17.5. E (1, 2, 3, and 4)
The simple columnar epithelium of the oviduct is composed of peg cells and ciliated cells. Peg cells secrete a material that aids in nourishing spermatozoa.

17.6. D (4)
The basal layer of the uterine endometrium is supplied by the straight arteries and contains the deeper portions of the uterine glands. Cells from these glands reepithelialize the endometrial surface after the functional layer (supplied by the helical arteries) has been sloughed.

17.7. B (1 and 3)
The uterine endometrium undergoes hormonally regulated cyclic alterations. The phases are follicular, luteal, and menstrual. Active and resting refer to the phases characteristic of the mammary glands.

17.8. C (2 and 4)
The primary villi of the chorion are composed of a core of cytotrophoblasts surrounded by syncytiotrophoblasts. Extraembryonic mesenchyme is found in secondary villi and blood vessels are found in chorionic (tertiary) villi.

17.9. C
The fetal portion of the placenta consists of the chorionic plate. All other statements refer to the maternal portion of the placenta.

17.10. D
The mucosa of the vagina is lined by a stratified squamous nonkeratinized epithelium whose cells release glycogen. The normal bacterial flora of the vagina utilizes the glycogen to manufacture lactic acid.

17.11. E
The only incorrect statement is that the mammary gland forms alveoli only during menstruation. Alveoli are formed only during pregnancy.

For **17.12** to **17.15**, refer to Figure 17.11, a section of a graafian follicle.

17.12. E, theca interna

17.13. B, liquor folliculi

17.14. D, membrana granulosa

17.15. B, antrum

18
Male Reproductive System

Male Reproductive System

—consists of the testes contained in the scrotum, the genital ducts and their associated glands (accessory glands), and the penis.

—testes function to produce spermatozoa (sperm) and to synthesize the hormone testosterone.

—major accessory glands include the paired seminal vesicles and the single prostate gland.

—minor accessory glands include the two bulbourethral glands located at the root of the penis.

—accessory glands function to manufacture the fluid portion of the semen, which transports and nourishes the spermatozoa as they pass through the excretory ducts.

—penis is the male copulatory organ that delivers spermatozoa into the female reproductive tract and serves as a conduit for excretion of urine from the body.

Testes

Testis

—is an ovoid body, about 4 to 5 cm long, that is housed within the scrotum.

—develops retroperitoneally in the abdominal cavity and then descends into the scrotum, carrying parietal and visceral layers of the peritoneum (the tunica vaginalis) that partially cover the testis on its anterior and lateral surfaces.

Tunica Albuginea

—is the thick fibrous connective tissue capsule of the testis.

—is thickened posteriorly to form the mediastinum testis from which connective tissue septa arise to divide the organ into approximately 250 compartments (lobuli testis).

Lobuli Testis

—are pyramidal-shaped incomplete compartments that intercommunicate.

—contain from 1 to 4 seminiferous tubules each, embedded in a meshwork of loose connective tissue where nerves, vessels, and scattered interstitial cells of Leydig are present.

Figure 18.1. Diagram of the male reproductive system. **A,** testis; **B,** head of the epididymis; **C,** spermatic cord; **D,** penis; **E,** glans penis; **1,** tunica albuginea; **2,** septum testis; **3,** seminiferous tubule; **4,** mediastinum and rete testis; **5,** ductuli efferentes; **6,** ductus epididymis; **7,** ductus deferens; **8,** seminal vesicle; **9,** ampulla of ductus deferens; **10,** prostate gland; **11,** ejaculatory duct; **12,** colliculus seminalis; **13–16,** prostatic, membranous, and penile portions of the urethra. (From Kelly DE, Wood RL, Enders AC: *Bailey's Textbook of Microscopic Anatomy*, ed 18. Baltimore, Williams & Wilkins, 1984.)

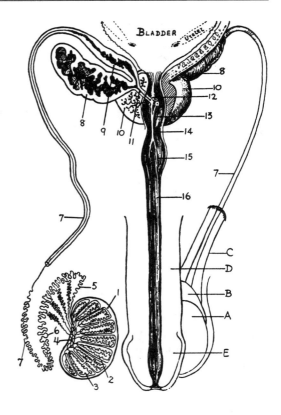

Interstitial Cells of Leydig

—are located in the interstitial spaces between the seminiferous tubules.

—mature and begin to secrete during puberty and are richly supplied with capillaries and lymphatic vessels.

—are round to polygonal in shape, possess a large central nucleus, many mitochondria, a well-developed Golgi apparatus, and many lipid droplets.

—are endocrine cells that produce the male sex hormone testosterone, when stimulated by luteinizing hormone (interstitial cell stimulating hormone) from the pituitary gland.

Seminiferous Tubules

—are the sites where spermatozoa are produced.

—are 30 to 70 cm long, with a diameter of 150 to 250 μm.

—are lined by a complex, stratified epithelium.

—are enveloped by a fibrous connective tissue tunic, composed of several layers of fibroblasts. Myoid cells, resembling smooth muscle, are present in the inner layer of some species, but not in humans.

—form tortuous pathways through the organ before they become continuous with the short straight tubuli recti.

Tubuli Recti

—have a narrow lumen lined by a simple cuboidal epithelium.

—lead into the rete testis, a network of epithelial-lined channels located in the mediastinum.

Vein   Thickened basement membrane

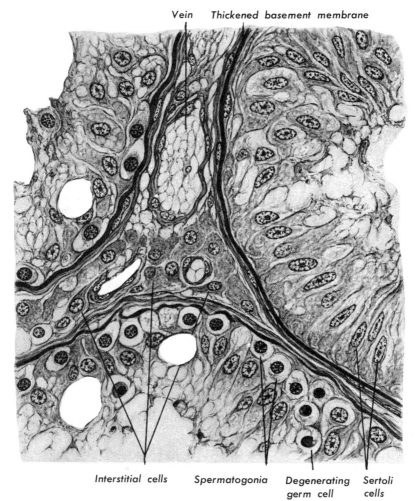

Interstitial cells   Spermatogonia   Degenerating   Sertoli
germ cell   cells

Figure 18.2. Drawing of interstitial cells of Leydig located between three sections of seminiferous tubules. (From Copenhaver WM, Bunge RP, Bunge MB: *Bailey's Textbook of Histology*, ed 16. Baltimore, Williams & Wilkins, 1971.)

Ductuli Efferentes
—lead from the rete testis into the epididymis.

Seminiferous Epithelium
—is composed of two different types of cells, the spermatogenic cells from which the germ cells eventually develop and the Sertoli cells, which support and provide nutrition to the spermatogenic cells.
—is 4 to 8 cell layers thick.

Sertoli Cells
—are columnar, extremely complex in shape, and extend from the basal lamina to the lumen.
—their apical and lateral plasma membranes are markedly irregular in outline since they envelop the developing germ cells.

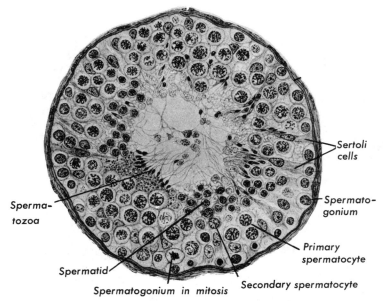

Figure 18.3. Drawing of a cross section of a seminiferous tubule. (From Kelly DE, Wood RL, Enders AC: *Bailey's Textbook of Microscopic Anatomy*, ed 18. Baltimore, Williams & Wilkins, 1984.)

—contain a well-developed smooth endoplasmic reticulum, some rough endoplasmic reticulum, an abundance of mitochondria and lysosomes, and an extensive Golgi apparatus.

—nucleus is pale, oval, displaying frequent indentations and a large nucleolus.

—form occluding junctions with adjoining Sertoli cells, thus subdividing the lumen of the seminiferous tubule into a basal and an adluminal compartment.

—zonulae occludentes are responsible for establishing the blood-testis barrier that serves to protect the developing sperm cells from autoimmune reactions.

Functions

—of Sertoli cells are manifold.

—support, protect, and nourish developing spermatozoa.

—phagocytose excess cytoplasm discarded by spermatids in the process of spermiogenesis.

—secrete a fluid into the seminiferous tubules that transports spermatozoa to the genital ducts.

—contain FSH receptors and under FSH influence synthesize androgen-binding protein (ABP) that binds testosterone, concentrating it to permit sperm maturation.

—secrete inhibin, a hormone that inhibits synthesis and release of FSH from the anterior pituitary.

Spermatogenic Cells

—include several characteristic cell types in the seminiferous epithelium: spermatogonia, primary spermatocytes, secondary spermatocytes, spermatids, and spermatozoa.

—each of these cells represents a dinstinct stage in the differentiation of male germ cells. The entire process is known as spermatogenesis.

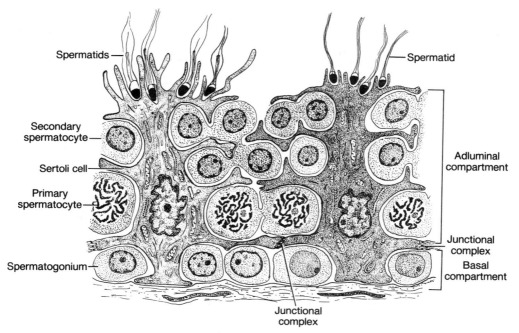

Figure 18.4. Drawing of the germinal epithelium. (From Krause WJ, Cutts JH: *Concise Text of Histology*, ed 2. Baltimore, Williams & Wilkins, 1986.)

Spermatogenesis

—is divided into three phases: spermatocytogenesis, meiosis, and spermiogenesis.

—in man takes approximately 64 days; its cell divisions are unusual, in that the daughter cells remain connected to each other via intercellular bridges (forming a syncytium).

Syncytium

—may be responsible for the synchronous development of germ cells along any one seminiferous tubule.

—is disrupted at the completion of spermatogenesis, when the individual spermatozoa are released into the lumen.

Spermatocytogenesis

—refers to division of the spermatogonia to provide a continuous supply of cells that will give rise to primary spermatocytes.

Meiosis

—is two successive divisions that reduce the chromosome number from diploid to haploid and produce spermatids.

Spermiogenesis

—is cytodifferentiation and transformation of spermatids to form spermatozoa.

Spermatogonia

—are the diploid germ cells that sit upon the basal lamina.

—are of three types: pale type A, dark type A, and type B.

Pale Type A

—are small (about 12 μm diameter) and possess a pale-staining nucleus and cytoplasm containing spherical mitochondria, a small Golgi complex, and abundant free ribosomes.

—at puberty these cells undergo mitosis and give rise to either more pale type A spermatogonia (to maintain the supply of spermatogonia) or type B spermatogonia (which undergo mitosis and give rise to primary spermatocytes).

Dark Type A

—(with dark nuclei) represent noncycling, reserve cells that have the potential to produce more pale type A cells.

Primary Spermatocytes

—are identified as the largest germ cells in the seminiferous epithelium.

—are diploid cells (46 chromosomes) that undergo meiosis.

Prophase

—of the first meiotic division is long (it takes more than 22 days).

—includes several stages: leptotene, zygotene, pachytene, diplotene (during which crossing over, the exchange of genetic material between homologous chromosomes, occurs), and diakinesis.

—is followed by metaphase I, anaphase I, and telophase I, which compose the first meiotic division.

First Meiotic Division

—results in the formation of small secondary spermatocytes.

Secondary Spermatocytes

—possess the haploid number of chromosomes (23), and the amount of DNA has been reduced (from 4N to 2N).

—quickly undergo the second meiotic division, producing spermatids.

Spermatids

—are haploid cells with 23 chromosomes and one-half the amount of DNA (since no S phase took place).

—are small (7 to 8 μm diameter) and located near the lumen of the seminiferous tubule.

—their nuclei often display regions of condensed chromatin.

—contain a pair of centrioles, mitochondria, free ribosomes, smooth endoplasmic reticulum, and a well-developed Golgi apparatus.

—undergo the cytodifferentiation process known as spermiogenesis.

Spermiogenesis

—is the unique differentiation process whereby spermatids transform into spermatozoa that are released into the lumen of the seminiferous tubule.

—acrosome and sperm tail are formed during spermiogenesis, the nucleus becomes condensed and elongated, and excess cytoplasm not directly involved in forming the spermatozoan is shed and phagocytosed by Sertoli cells.

—is divided into four phases: Golgi, cap, acrosome, and maturation phases.

Golgi Phase

—of spermiogenesis is characterized by the formation of proacrosomal granules in the Golgi complex.

Proacrosomal Granules

—coalesce to form a single acrosomal granule enclosed within an acrosomal vesicle, which becomes attached to the anterior end of the nuclear envelope.

Centrioles

—migrate away from the nucleus to form the flagellar axoneme and then retreat toward the nucleus and assist in forming the connecting piece associated with the tail.

Cap Phase

—involves the expansion of the acrosomal vesicle over much of the nucleus, to form the acrosomal cap.

Acrosomes

—contain hydrolytic enzymes (acid phosphatase, neuraminidase, hyaluronidase, protease, and phosphatase).

Acrosomal Reaction

—refers to the release of enzymes that facilitate the dissociation of the cells of the corona radiata and the digestion of the zona pellucida.

Acrosome Phase

—is characterized by the nucleus becoming condensed and flattened, mitochondria aggregating around the proximal portion of the flagellum to form the middle piece, and elongation of the spermatid.

Elongation

—may be facilitated by a cylinder of microtubules, the manchette. By the end of the acrosome phase the spermatids are oriented with their acrosomes pointing toward the base of the seminiferous tubule.

Maturation Phase

—is characterized by excess cytoplasm being discarded (including the intercellular bridges that connected the spermatids) and phagocytosed by Sertoli cells.
—is completed when nonmotile spermatozoa are released (tail first) into the lumen of the seminiferous tubule.

Cycle of Seminiferous Epithelium

—refers to the wave-like sequence of maturation that occurs along the seminiferous tubules.

One Cycle

—is the reappearance of identical cell associations within the epithelium.
—in humans is approximately 16 days, so that four cycles (64 days) must occur for a spermatogonium to be transformed into a spermatozoon.

Histophysiology

Temperature

—of 35°C is critical for the development of spermatozoa.

—is achieved in the scrotum by the pampiniform plexus of veins that wrap around the testicular artery and function to dissipate heat.

—is achieved also by evaporation of sweat from the skin of the scrotum.

—below 35°C, contraction of the cremaster muscle in the spermatic cord brings the testis close to the body wall to increase the temperature.

Cryptorchidism

—is a condition when the testes fail to descend into the scrotum during development.

—the normal body temperature inhibits spermatogenesis, resulting in sterility. However, this condition does not affect testosterone production.

Luteinizing Hormone (LH)

—of the pituitary gland stimulates the interstitial cells of Leydig to secrete testosterone, which is responsible for the normal development of male germ cells and secondary sex characteristics.

Follicle-Stimulation Hormone (FSH)

—of the pituitary gland acts on the Sertoli cells, promoting the synthesis of androgen-binding protein (ABP).

ABP

—binds with testosterone and maintains a high concentration of testosterone in the seminiferous tubules, where it is essential for spermatogenesis.

—binds estrogens and inhibits spermatogenesis. Increased testosterone levels inhibit LH release, whereas FSH release is stopped by inhibin (secreted by Sertoli cells).

Genital Ducts

—convey the spermatozoa and semen to outside of the body.

—extend from the seminiferous tubules to the urethra. Although they are continuous, they are structurally and histologically different. Their names identify the regional division and unique characteristics they possess.

Tubuli Recti

—are short straight tubules, located in the mediastinum testis, which convey spermatozoa from the seminiferous tubules to the rete testis.

—their lumen is lined by a simple cuboidal epithelium having cells that possess microvilli and a single flagellum on their luminal surface.

Rete Testis

—is a labyrinthine plexus of anastomosing channels within the mediastinum testis that connect the tubuli recti with the ductuli efferentes.

—are lined by a simple cuboidal epithelium, and, like those of the tubuli recti, many of the cells possess a single flagellum.

Ductuli Efferentes

—are a collection of 10 to 20 tubules leading from the rete testis to the ductus epididymis.

—are lined by a simple epithelium, composed of alternating clusters of (nonciliated) cuboidal and (ciliated) columnar cells.

Cuboidal Cells

—possess microvilli, contain lysosomal granules, and function to reabsorb fluid from the semen.

Ciliated Columnar Cells

—aid in transporting the nonmotile spermatozoa toward the epididymis.

Smooth Muscle

—in the form of a thin circular layer underlies the basal lamina surrounding the ductuli efferentes epithelium.

Ductus Epididymis

—begins as the terminal portions of the ductuli efferentes fuse.
—is a narrow, highly coiled tubule, 4 to 6 meters long.
—is surrounded by connective tissue containing blood vessels.
—is subdivided into a head, body, and tail region.
—its lumen is lined by pseudostratified columnar epithelium.

Epithelium

—is composed of basal and principal cells.

Basal Cells

—are round and appear undifferentiated, apparently serving as precursors of the columnar principal cells.

Principal Cells

—possess stereocilia (long irregular branching microvilli) on their luminal surface.
—also possess endoplasmic reticulum, a large Golgi complex, lysosomes, and many pinocytotic and coated vesicles in their apical portions (suggesting fluid resorption).
—secrete glycerophosphocholine, a substance that probably inhibits capacitation.

Capacitation

—is a process whereby the sperm becomes capable of fertilizing the ovum, and, although it begins in the epididymis, it is not completed until the sperm reaches the oviduct.

Basal Lamina

—supports the epithelium and is in turn surrounded by circular layers of smooth muscle, which increase in thickness and undergo peristaltic contractions that move the sperm toward the ductus deferens.

Ductus Deferens (vas deferens)

—begins at the end of the ductus epididymis as a straight tube with a thick muscular wall.

Pseudostratified Epithelium

—(with stereocilia) similar to that of the ductus epididymis, lines the narrow, irregular lumen of the ductus deferens.

Muscular Wall

—is composed of inner and outer layers of longitudinally oriented smooth muscle, separated from one another by a middle circular layer.

Ampulla

—is the dilated portion of the ductus deferens that leads directly to the prostate gland.
—its epithelium is thickened and greatly folded.
—its distal end receives the seminal vesicle, thus forming the ejaculatory duct that enters the prostate gland.

Ejaculatory Duct

—is the straight continuation of the ductus deferens beyond where it receives the ducts of the seminal vesicles.
—lacks a muscular wall. It enters the prostate gland and terminates as a slit on the colliculus seminalis, in the prostatic urethra.

Accessory Genital Glands

—include the seminal vesicles, the prostate gland, and the bulbourethral glands.
—produce most of the seminal fluid.

Seminal Vesicles

—are the paired tortuous tubular glands (15 cm in length) located adjacent the posterior aspect of the bladder.
—their ducts join the ductus deferens just prior to its entering the prostate gland.

Pseudostratified Columnar Epithelium

—lines the extensively folded mucosa of this gland.
—consists of low columnar cells interspersed with cuboidal basal cells (whose height is testosterone dependent).

Columnar Cells

—have many yellow lipochrome pigment granules and secretory granules, contain a large Golgi apparatus, many mitochondria, and an abundant rough endoplasmic reticulum.

Lamina Propria

—consists of fibroelastic connective tissue surrounded by an inner circular and an outer longitudinal layer of smooth muscle.

Adventitia

—is also composed of fibroelastic connective tissue.

Secretory Product

—is a yellow, viscous fluid that is rich in fructose and other substances and constitutes about 70% of the human ejaculate.

Prostate Gland

—surrounds the urethra as it exits the urinary bladder and is the largest accessory gland.
—consists of 30 to 50 discrete branched tubuloalveolar glands that empty their contents into the prostatic urethra (via excretory ducts).

Glands of the Prostate
—are arranged in three concentric layers (mucosal, submucosal, and main) around the urethra and are surrounded by a fibroelastic capsule that contains smooth muscle.
—stroma from the capsule penetrate the gland and divide it into lobes.

Simple or Pseudostratified Columnar Epithelium
—lines the glands, and the fibroelastic connective tissue enveloping them contains elastic fibers and is richly vascularized.

Epithelial Cells
—contain abundant rough endoplasmic reticulum, a well-developed large Golgi complex, numerous lysosomes, and many secretory granules.

Prostatic Concretions
—composed of glycoprotein are sometimes observed in the lumina of the glands.
—may become calcified and their numbers increase with age.

Secretion
—of the prostate, under the influence of dihydrotestosterone, is a whitish, thin fluid containing proteolytic enzymes, citric acid, acid phosphatase, and lipids.

Prostatic Carcinoma
—induces elevated acid phosphatase blood levels, which is used as a diagnostic tool.

Bulbourethral Glands (Cowper's glands)
—located adjacent to the membraneous urethra, empty their clear secretion into the lumen to lubricate it.
—are lined by a simple cuboidal or columnar epithelium. Wide fibroelastic septa (containing smooth and skeletal muscle cells) extend from the capsule to subdivide the gland into lobules.

Penis
—functions both as an execretory organ for urine and as a copulatory organ for delivering sperm into the female reproductive tract.
—is composed of three cylindrical masses of erectile tissue. The paired corpora cavernosa lie dorsally and the single corpus spongiosum contains the penile (spongy) urethra.
—is covered by skin that overlies a loose connective tissue sheath that surrounds the corpora cavernosa and corpus spongiosum.
—skin (distally) lacks hair follicles and contains only a few sweat glands.
—hypodermis contains a prominent layer of smooth muscle but no adipose tissue.

Prepuce
—that portion of skin that covers the glans penis.
—resembles a mucous membrane, since it is lined by stratified squamous nonkeratinized epithelium.

Tunica Albuginea
—is the thick fibrous connective tissue sheath surrounding the three erectile bodies.

Figure 18.5. Cross section of the penis. (From Krause WJ, Cutts JH: *Concise Text of Histology*, ed 2. Baltimore, Williams & Wilkins, 1986.)

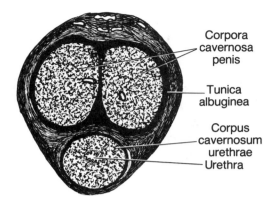

The arrangement of the dense collagen bundles in the tunica permit extensibility of the penis during erection.

Corpora Cavernosa

—are the two paired erectile bodies located dorsally in the penis.
—contain irregular vascular spaces lined by a continuous layer of endothelial cells separated from each other by trabeculae of connective tissue and smooth muscle cells.

Vascular Spaces

—are decreased in size toward the periphery of the corpora.
—become engorged with blood during erection, making the penis turgid.

Corpus Spongiosum

—is the singular erectile body surrounding the spongy urethra.
—its erectile tissue is similar to those of the corpora cavernosa, except that the trabeculae contain more elastic fibers and only a few smooth muscle cells.
—its vascular spaces are uniform throughout.

Glands of Littrè

—are mucus-secreting glands that are also present throughout the length of the penile urethra.

Glans Penis

—is the terminal end of the corpus spongiosum.
—contains dense connective tissue and longitudinal muscle fibers.

Erection

—occurs when the erectile tissues become distended with blood due to parasympathetic stimulation mediated by tactile or erotic stimulation.

Parasympathetic Impulses

—constrict arteriovenous shunts and dilate the helicine arteries, which force blood into the spaces of the erectile bodies under pressure, engorging them with blood.

Ejaculation

—and/or termination of erotic stimulation causes diminished parasympathetic activity, followed by detumescence, and the penis returns to the flaccid state.

REVIEW TESTS
MALE REPRODUCTIVE SYSTEM

DIRECTIONS: *One* or *more* of the given statements or completions is/are correct. Choose answer:

A. if only **1**, **2**, and **3** are correct
B. if only **1** and **3** are correct
C. if only **2** and **4** are correct
D. if only **4** is correct
E. if **all** are correct

18.1. The testis
1. is subdivided into lobules by connective tissue septa, derived from the tunica albuginea
2. manufactures androgens
3. contains seminiferous tubules
4. is partially covered by the tunica vaginalis

18.2. Seminiferous tubules
1. have a tortuous course in the lobuli testis
2. do not receive seminal fluid from the rete testis
3. possess two different populations of cells in the epithelium
4. possess a skeletal muscle layer in its tunica propria

18.3. Interstitial cells of Leydig
1. become functional at puberty
2. are located within the seminiferous tubules
3. are stimulated by luteinizing hormone
4. secrete much of the fluid portion of semen

18.4. Type B spermatogonia
1. are germ cells that develop from secondary spermatocytes
2. undergo mitotic activity subsequent to sexual maturity
3. develop through meiotic divisions
4. give rise to primary spermatocytes

18.5. The ductus epididymis
1. begins at the distal terminals of the ductuli efferentes
2. is lined by a pseudostratified columnar epithelium
3. reabsorbs fluid from its lumen
4. secretes glycerophosphocholine, a substance that inhibits capacitation of spermatozoa

DIRECTIONS: Each of the following questions contains five suggested completions. Choose the *one* that is *best* in each case.

18.6. Testosterone is produced by
A. interstitial cells of Leydig
B. Sertoli cells
C. spermatogonia
D. spermatids
E. spermatocytes

18.7. Seminiferous tubules join the rete testis via the
A. epididymis
B. tubuli recti
C. ductuli efferentes
D. ductus deferens
E. none of the above

18.8. Spermiogenesis includes all of the following stages *except*
A. meiosis I phase
B. maturation phase
C. Golgi phase
D. cap phase
E. acrosome phase

18.9. The ductus deferens can best be identified by
A. a smooth bore lumen
B. three separate muscle coats
C. transitional epithelium
D. flattened mucosa

18.10. The accessory genital gland whose secretion is responsible for lubricating the urethra is the
A. prostate gland
B. bulbourethral glands
C. seminal vesicles
D. none of the above

DIRECTIONS: The following questions or statements refer to the drawing below (Fig. 18.6). The letters on the figure are answers to the numbered items appearing below the drawing. For each numbered item select the *one* letter that *best* corresponds to that item. Each letter may be used once, more than once, or not at all.

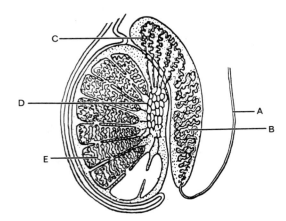

Figure 18.6.

18.11. seminiferous tubule

18.12. ductuli efferentes

18.13. ductus deferens

18.14. ductus epididymis

18.15. tubuli recti

ANSWERS AND EXPLANATIONS

MALE REPRODUCTIVE SYSTEM

18.1. E (all are correct)

The capsule of the testis, the tunica albuginea (which is partly invested by the tunica vaginalis) sends septa into the organ, dividing it into about 250 lobuli testis. Each lobule contains about 3 to 4 seminiferous tubules. Interstitial cells of Leydig manufacture the androgen testosterone.

18.2. A (1, 2, and 3)

Seminiferous tubules, which do not receive seminal fluid from the rete testis, begin as branched or blind ends and have a tortuous course within the lobuli testis. The epithelium of the seminiferous tubules has two distinct populations of cells, spermatogenic and Sertoli. There are no skeletal muscles associated with the seminiferous tubules.

18.3. B (1 and 3)

Interstitial cells of Leydig, located in the interstitium between the seminiferous tubules, do not become functional until after puberty, when they are stimulated by luteinizing hormone to secrete testosterone.

18.4. C (2 and 4)

Type B spermatogonia are germ cells that undergo mitotic activity subsequent to sexual maturity and give rise to primary spermatocytes.

18.5. E (all are correct)

The ductus epididymis begins at the distal terminals of the ductuli efferentes and is lined by a pseudostratified columnar epithelium. These columnar cells resorb fluid from the lumen. Additionally, the ductus epididymis secretes glycerophosphocholine, which functions to inhibit capacitation of the spermatozoa.

18.6. A

Testosterone is produced by the interstitial cells of Leydig. Sertoli cells are the supporting cells of the seminiferous epithelium. Spermatogonia are the germ cells that give rise to the cells that eventually differentiate into spermatids and finally into spermatozoa.

18.7. B

Seminiferous tubules that lie in the lobuli testis join the rete testis via short straight tubes called tubuli recti. Ductuli efferentes drain the rete testis and their distal ends fuse to give rise to the ductus epididymis.

18.8. A

Spermiogenesis is the process whereby spermatids differentiate into spermatozoa. This process includes the Golgi phase, cap phase, acrosome phase, and maturation phase. Meiosis I has occurred prior to spermiogenesis and plays no part in this process.

18.9. B

One of the major identifying characteristics of the ductus deferens is that it possesses a thick muscular wall consisting of inner and outer longitudinal muscle layers separated by a circular muscular layer. The lumen is lined by pseudostratified columnar epithelium. The mucosa is irregular and folded.

18.10. B

Bulbourethral glands (Cowper's glands), located adjacent the membranous urethra, secrete a lubricating fluid into the urethra. The prostate gland secretes a fluid containing proteolytic enzymes, acid phosphatase, citric acid, and lipids. The seminal vesicles secrete most of the seminal fluid.

18.11. E, seminiferous tubule

18.12. C, ductuli efferentes

18.13. A, ductus deferens

18.14. B, ductus epididymis

18.15. D, tubuli recti

19

Special Senses

Special Senses

—included in special senses:

—taste buds, which are chemoreceptors located in the oral cavity (discussed in Chapter 13).

—olfactory organs, chemoreceptors located in the nasal cavity that perceive odors (discussed in Chapter 12).

—eyes, the photoreceptor system responsible for vision.

—ears, audioreceptors responsible for hearing.

—other types of receptors located in the skin, fascia, muscles, joints, and tendons are specialized to receive stimuli from only one of the following modalities: pressure, temperature, vibration, pain, and proprioception. The muscle-tendon proprioceptor system is discussed in Chapter 6.

Specialized Receptors

—are divided morphologically into free nerve terminals and encapsulated nerve endings (ensheathed in a connective tissue capsule).

—represent dendritic nerve endings responsible for receiving stimuli related to pain, touch and pressure, and temperature.

—usually act to receive only one sensory modality (adequate stimulus); most receptors respond to excessive stimuli from other modalities.

Touch and Pressure

Pacinian Corpuscles

—are large ellipsoid (1 to 4 mm diameter) encapsulated receptors located in the dermis and hypodermis.

—are abundant in the digits and breasts and in the connective tissue of the mesenteries and joints.

—resemble an onion since they are composed of a multilayered capsule of fibroblasts, collagen, and tissue fluid, surrounding a core of unmyelinated nerve terminal.

—respond to pressure, touch, and vibration.

Ruffini's Endings

—are encapsulated receptors (0.2 to 1 mm) located in the dermis and in joints.

—are composed of groups of branched terminals (from myelinated fibers) that are surrounded by a thin connective tissue capsule.

—function in pressure and touch reception.

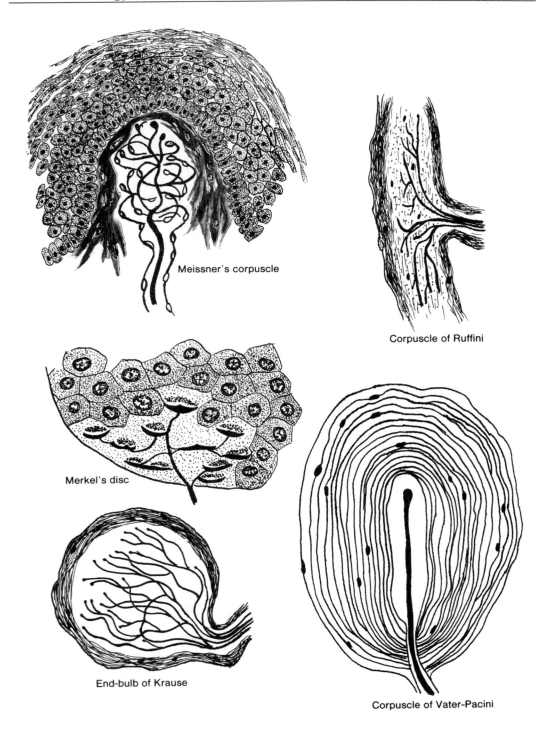

Figure 19.1. Diagram of the various types of encapsulated nerve endings. (From Krause WJ, Cutts JH: *Concise Text of Histology*, ed 2. Baltimore, Williams & Wilkins, 1985.)

Meissner's Corpuscles

—are encapsulated ellipsoid receptors (about $150 \times 40 \ \mu m$) located in the dermal papilla of thick skin as well as in the skin of the eyelids, lips, and nipples.

—connective tissue capsule envelops the nerve terminal and its associated Schwann cells.

—function in fine touch reception.

Free Nerve Endings

—are unencapsulated, unmyelinated terminations located in the skin, usually surrounding hair follicles.

—are arranged in longitudinal and circular arrays around most of the follicle.

—function in touch reception.

Cold, Heat, and Pain

Cold Receptors

—(25° to 30°C) are nerve endings from thin myelinated nerve fibers.

—enter the epidermis, lose their myelin and Schwann cell cytoplasm, branch, and terminate among the deeper cells in the epidermis.

Heat Receptors

—(40° to 42°C) located in the same areas are also unmyelinated.

Pain Receptors (nociceptors)

—are delicate myelinated fibers that lose their myelin prior to entering the epidermis.

—branch extensively and give rise to endings containing many clear vesicles and some large dense-cored vesicles.

Eye

Eye (orb; globe)

—is the visual organ located in the bony orbit of the skull. Light passing through the cornea is focused on the retina, where specialized cells encode the various patterns of the image for transmission to the brain via the optic nerve.

—possesses intrinsic muscles that function *1)* to adjust the aperature of the iris and *2)* to alter the lens diameter, permitting accommodation for close vision.

—its anterior surface is moistened with lacrimal fluid (tears) secreted by the lacrimal gland.

Upper and Lower Eyelids

—cover and protect the anterior surface.

Extrinsic Muscles

—attached to the external aspect of the globe move the eyes in a coordinated manner to access the desired visual fields.

Orb

—is composed of three tunics: sclera, vascular layer, and retina.

Sclera

—possesses an outer fibrous layer that maintains the shape and serves as an attachment site for the extrinsic muscles.

—its anterior aspect is transparent and is known as the cornea.

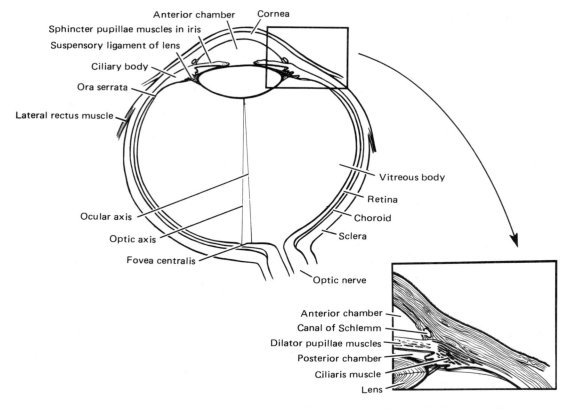

Figure 19.2. Diagram of the internal anatomy of the orb. (From Hiatt JL, Gartner LP: *Textbook of Head and Neck Anatomy*, ed 2. Baltimore, Williams & Wilkins, 1987.)

Middle Vascular Tunic
—is composed of the iris, ciliary body, and the pigmented choroid.

Retina
—is the inner layer that contains the photoreceptor cells responsible for generating impulses that are transmitted (via the optic nerve) to the brain.

Refractive Media
—include the aqueous humor, the vitreous body, and the lens.

Tunica Fibrosa
—(external layer of the orb) is composed of the sclera (white of the eye) posteriorly and the transparent cornea anteriorly.

Sclera
—is the relatively avascular, tough connective tissue that covers the posterior five-sixths of the orb.
—is composed of interlacing collagen bundles arranged parallel to the surface of the globe.
—its external surface (episclera) receives insertion of the extrinsic ocular muscles and is loosely attached via thin collagen fibers to Tenon's capsule.

—space between Tenon's capsule and the sclera permits the eyeball to rotate freely and change the visual fields.

Cornea

—is the transparent, highly innervated, avascular anterior one-sixth of the tunica fibrosa whose junction with the sclera is marked by the limbus.
—receives metabolites from the vessels in the vascular limbus.
—is composed of five layers: epithelium, Bowman's membrane, stroma, Descemet's membrane, and endothelium.

Corenal Epithelium

—is classified as stratified squamous nonkeratinized epithelium, five to six cell layers thick.
—its superficial layer possesses microvilli that trap moisture, protecting the cornea from dehydration.

Bowman's Membrane

—is the homogenous noncellular layer (7 to 12 μm thick) composed of compact interlacing collagen fibers and intercellular substances, which function to provide form, stability, and strength to the cornea.

Stroma

—is the thickest layer of the cornea, formed by many layers of collagen bundles arranged at right angles to each other.
—extensions of fibroblasts intermingle among these fibers and are bathed in an amorphous glycoprotein substance rich in chondroitin sulfate.
—channels located in the region of the limbus are lined by endothelium, forming the canal of Schlemm.

Canal of Schlemm

—drains fluid from the anterior chamber of the eye into the venous system.

Descemet's Membrane

—is a thick (5 to 10 μm) basal lamina separating the stroma from the endothelium lining the cornea.
—is manufactured by this endothelium.

Endothelium

—lining the posterior aspect of the cornea is composed of simple squamous cells exhibiting numerous pinocytotic vesicles.
—its cells continually resorb fluid from the stroma and thus contribute to the transparency of the cornea.

Tunica Vasculosa (uvea)

—is the middle layer of the eye whose three parts are the choroid, the ciliary body, and the iris.

Choroid

—is the highly vascular, pigmented layer of the eye.
—is loosely attached to the tunica fibrosa.
—its loose connective tissue contains many melanocytes.

Choriocapillary Layer

—is the deep (fenestrated) capillary layer of the choroid.

—provides nourishment to the retina and is separated from it by Bruch's membrane.

Bruch's Membrane

—is a thin hyaline structure that extends from the optic disk (exit site of optic nerve) to the ora serrata (anterior termination of the optic retina).

—is composed of a central core of elastic fibers sandwiched between collagen fibers that are bordered on one side by basal lamina from the endothelial cells and on the other side by basal lamina of the pigment epithelium.

Ciliary Body

—completely encircles the lens and is the region of the vascular tunic located between the ora serrata and the iris.

—is wedge-shaped and composed of loose connective tissue rich in elastic fibers, melanocytes, and blood vessels surrounding the ciliary muscle.

—its inner surface is lined by two layers of cells, an outer columnar layer rich in melanin and an inner nonpigmented simple columnar epithelium.

Ciliary Processes

—are approximately 70 radially arranged extensions of the ciliary body.

—their connective tissue core has many fenestrated capillaries, and their surfaces are covered by two epithelial layers.

Unpigmented Inner Layer

—of epithelial cells transports components from the plasma in the posterior chamber and thus forms the aqueous humor.

Suspensory Ligaments (zonule)

—arise from the ciliary processes and insert into the capsule of the lens, serving to anchor it in place.

Ciliary Muscle

—is grouped into three bundles.

—is attached to the sclera and ciliary body in such a manner that its contractions stretch the choroid body and release tension on the suspensory ligament and lens.

—when it contracts, permits the lens to become more convex, thereby accommodating the eye to focus on nearby objects.

Aqueous Humor

—is a plasma-like fluid formed by epithelial cells lining the ciliary processes.

—is secreted into the posterior chamber of the eye and flows to the anterior chamber by passing between the lens and the iris.

—upon reaching the anterior chamber, flows into the canal of Schlemm and from there into the venous system.

Glaucoma

—is caused by an increase in intraocular pressure due to obstructions that prevent drainage of aqueous humor from the eye.

Iris

—is the most anterior extension of the choroid, separating the anterior and posterior chambers from one another.

—incompletely covers the anterior surface of the lens, forming an adjustable opening, the pupil.
—its anterior surface is covered by an incomplete layer of pigment cells and fibroblasts.
—its wall is composed of loose, vascular connective tissue containing melanocytes and fibroblasts.
—its deep surface is covered by a two-layered epithelium with pigmented cells, which blocks light from entering the interior of the eye, except via the pupil.

Eye Color
—is a function of the number of melanocytes in the stroma of the iris.
—if only a few melanocytes are present, the eyes are blue.
—increasing amounts of pigment impart darker colors to the eye.

Dilatator Pupillae Muscle
—is composed of myoepithelial cells and is responsible for dilating the pupil.
—muscle fibers radiate from the periphery of the iris toward the pupil.
—when it contracts, due to stimulation by sympathetic nerve fibers, the pupil dilates.

Sphincter Pupillae Muscle
—is the smooth muscle located in the iris.
—is arranged in concentric rings around the pupillary orifice, and when it contracts, due to innervation by parasympathetic nerve fibers, the pupil constricts.

Lens
—is a biconvex, transparent, flexible structure located directly behind the iris.
—is held in place by the zonule fibers from the suspensory ligament that arises from the ciliary body and inserts upon the margins (equator) of the lens.
—consists of three parts: the lens capsule, the subcapsular epithelium, and lens fibers.

Lens Capsule
—is a thick (10 to 20 μm) carbohydrate-rich coating that envelops the lens epithelium.
—is a basement membrane, manufactured by the underlying anterior epithelial cells and lens fibers.

Subcapsular Epithelium
—is located only on the anterior surface.
—is composed of a single layer of cuboidal cells that communicate with each other via gap junctions.
—its cells interdigitate with lens fibers, especially at the equator, where the epithelial cells become more elongated.

Lens Fibers
—represent highly differentiated, elongated cells filled with a group of proteins called crystallins.
—differentiate from the subcapsular epithelium (at the level of the equator).
—mature lens fibers lack both nuclei and organelles.
—new lens fibers are added at the equator, but this function diminishes with increasing age.

Suspensory Ligament
—stretching between the lens and the ciliary body keeps tension on the lens, enabling it to focus on distant objects.

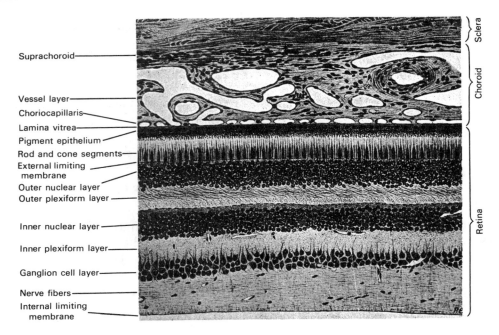

Figure 19.3. Drawing of a transverse section through the retina, sclera, and choroid. (From Copenhaver WM, Kelly DE, Wood RL: *Bailey's Textbook of Histology*, ed 17. Baltimore, Williams & Wilkins, 1978.)

Accommodation
—is the focus on close objects.
—is a function of the ciliary muscle, whose contraction pulls the choroid body anteriorly, releasing the tension on the lens and permitting it to become thicker, thus facilitating focusing on close objects.
—is gradually lost with advancing age due to the loss of elasticity in the lens.

Cataract
—is a condition where the lens becomes opaque. The vision becomes impaired and pigments or other substances can accumulate in the lens fibers, further debilitating vision.

Vitreous Body
—is the refractile gel filling the interior of the globe posterior to the lens.
—is composed mostly of water, collagen, and hyaluronic acid.

Retina
—is the innermost layer of the three tunics of the eye and is responsible for photoreception.
—develops initially as the optic vesicle (from the prosencephalon of the brain), which subsequently invaginates to form a two-layered optic cup, the pigmented layer and the neural retina. Its attachment stalk develops into the optic nerve.

Pigmented Layer of the Retina
—is the outer layer of the bilaminar optic cup.

Neural Retina

—is the inner layer of the retina responsible for photoreception.

Layers of the Retina

—are complex and are 10 in number. They are (from the outside inward) the *1*) pigment epithelium, *2*) layer of rods and cones, *3*) external limiting membrane, *4*) outer nuclear layer, *5*) outer plexiform layer, *6*) inner nuclear layer, *7*) inner plexiform layer, *8*) ganglion cell layer, *9*) optic nerve fiber layer, and *10*) inner limiting membrane.

Pigment Layer

Pigment Epithelium

—consists of a layer of columnar cells firmly attached to Bruch's membrane, the basement membrane separating the choroid from the retinal layer.

Cells of the Pigment Epithelium

—exhibit basal invaginations that contain basally located mitochondria, suggesting their involvement in ion transport.
—their cytoplasm contains smooth endoplasmic reticulum, and melanin granules are located apically and in their processes.
—melanin, synthesized by the pigment cells, absorbs light after the rods and cones have been stimulated.
—true junctional complexes (zonulae occludentes, zonulae adherentes, desmosomes, and gap junctions) attach the lateral borders of these cells together.
—microvilli and cylindrical sheaths extend from the apices of the pigment epithelial cells and invest the tips of the rods and cones.
—function in esterification and the transport of vitamin A to the rods and cones (which is necessary for visual pigment formation).
—phagocytose the shed tips of the outer segment of rods, and they absorb light.

Detachment of the Retina

—occurs when the neural and pigmented retinae become separated from each other.

Layer of Rods and Cones

Rods and Cones

—(photoreceptor cells) are neurons.
—their specialized dendrites, in the shape of either a rod or a cone, interdigitate with cells of the pigmented epithelium.
—their bases form a synaptic contact with cells of the bipolar layer.
—are described as having outer and inner segments, a nuclear region, and a synaptic region.

Outer Segments

—consist of stacks of flattened saccules filled with photosensitive pigment and arise from cilia that become highly modified.

Rods

—number about 120 million in each human retina.
—are long slender cells (50 μm in length) containing hundreds of stacks of flat membranous disks in their outer segment.

Disks

—are not continuous with the plasma membrane of the rod cell.

Constriction

—separates the outer and inner segments and contains an incomplete cilium (without the central two singlet microtubules) that terminates in a basal body within the inner segment.

Inner Segment

—possesses mitochondria, glycogen, and polyribosomes.

—produces proteins that migrate to the outer segment, where they become incorporated into the membranes of the disks.

Disks

—are eventually shed and are subsequently phagocytosed by the pigment epithelium.

Rods

—contain rhodopsin and are the receptors sensitive to light of low intensity.

—their outer segments face the back of the eye so that light must pass through the outer layers of the retina before reaching the photosensitive region of these cells.

—may synapse with a bipolar cell (giving rise to summation).

Rhodopsin

—is composed of opsins, the integral transmembrane proteins, to which retinal, the aldehyde form of vitamin A, is bound.

Light

—interacts with rhodopsin in the membranous disks of the rod outer segment, and retinal becomes dissociated from opsins (bleaching), which permits the diffusion of bound calcium from the disks into the cytoplasm of the outer segment.

Excess Ca^{2+}

—acts to hyperpolarize the cell by inhibiting the entrance of Na^+ into the cell (closing Na^+ channels).

Ionic Alterations

—generate electrical activity in the entire cell, which is relayed to other cells via gap junctions.

Reassembly

—of retinal and opsins is an active process in which Müller and pigment epithelial cells also participate.

—is accompanied by the recapture of calcium ions by the membranous disks, with subsequent reopening of Na^+ channels, and a reestablishment of the normal resting membrane potential.

Cones

—number about 6 million in the human retina. They are long, slender, photoreceptor cells (60 μm in length) similar to rods, except for a cone-shaped outer segment.

—possess membranous disks (invaginations of the plasma membrane).

—synthesize proteins in the inner segment. These proteins are passed to the entire outer segment, rather than being added to the newest disks (as in rods).

—contain iodopsin (photopigment).

—are sensitive to bright light and synapse individually with the bipolar cell.

—produce a greater visual acuity than do the rod cells.

Iodopsin

—is the photopigment contained in the disks of the cone outer segments.

—is located in different amounts in various types of cones, making the cone most sensitive either to the red, green, or blue region of the visual spectrum, thus accounting for the three types of cones.

External Limiting Membrane

—is a region characterized by junctional specializations (zonulae adherentes) between Müller (glial) cells and the rods and cones.

—many microvilli from the Müller cells project into this area.

—cone nuclei are usually located near the external limiting membrane.

Outer Nuclear Layer

—represents the area of the retina where the nuclei of the rods and cones are located.

Outer Plexiform Layer

—is a region where synapses occur between the axons of the photoreceptor cells and the bipolar and horizontal cells.

Synaptic Ribbons

—are observed within the rod and cone cells at these synapses.

Bipolar Cells

—relay stimuli from the rods and cones to the ganglion cells (third-order neurons).

Horizontal Cells

—synapse with numerous rods and cones (in a lateral fashion).

Inner Nuclear Layer

—contains the nuclei of bipolar cells and horizontal cells in addition to Müller, amacrine, and interplexiform cells.

Inner Plexiform Layers

—is the region of the retina where synapses occur between the axons of bipolar cells and the dendrites of ganglion cells.

—is the site of location of Müller and amacrine cell processes. The amacrine cells function to connect bipolar cells with ganglion cells.

Ganglion Cell Layer

—contains the ganglion cells, which synapse with bipolar cells and amacrine cells in the inner plexiform layer.

—cells of this layer are the final link in the retina's neural chain, and their collected axons become the fibers comprising the optic nerve.

—several types of ganglion cells are classified according to the shape of their dendrites.

Midget Ganglion Cells

—are the most common.

—possess a single dendrite.

Diffuse Ganglion Cells

—are multidendritic.

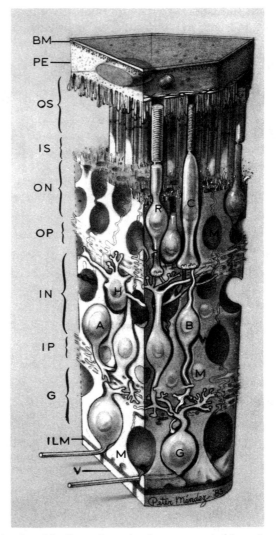

Figure 19.4. Schematic drawing of the three-dimensional arrangement of the cells comprising the retina. (From Kelly DE, Wood RL, Enders AC: *Bailey's Textbook of Microscopic Anatomy*, ed 18. Baltimore, Williams & Wilkins, 1984.)

Stratified Ganglion Cells

—contain an arborized dendritic process.

Hyperpolarization of the Rods and Cones

—activate ganglion cells (via horizontal and amacrine cells), which generate an action potential that reaches the visual relay system of the brain.

Optic Nerve Fiber Layer

—consists of the unmyelinated axons of ganglion cells, which form the fibers of the optic nerve.

—also contain Müller cell processes, glial cells, and blood vessels.

—at the optic disk each fiber pierces the sclera and acquires a myelin sheath.

Inner Limiting Membrane

—represents termination of the Müller cell processes and their associated basement membranes.

Fovea

—is a shallow depression in the posterior wall of the retina containing only cones.
—is the region of greatest visual activity.

Accessory Structures of the Eye

Conjunctiva

—is a transparent mucous membrane that lines the eyelids and is reflected onto the anterior portion of the orb up to the cornea, where it becomes continuous with the corneal epithelium.
—is composed of stratified columnar epithelium (having many goblet cells) lying on a basal lamina and separated from a lamina propria consisting of loose connective tissue.

Eyelids

—are folds of tissue that protect the eye.
—are covered by skin externally and lined by conjunctiva internally.
—contain three types of glands.
—their free margins display eyelashes.

Skin

—is elastic and covers a supportive framework of tarsal plates (dense fibroelastic connective tissue).

Tarsal Plates

—converge to form the medial and lateral palpebral ligaments, which attach to the orbital bones.

Orbicularis Oculi

—is the circular skeletal muscle that functions to close the eye. The orbital septum is the fascia that separates the orbicularis oculi from the eye proper.

Levator Palpebrae Superioris

—is a skeletal muscle that originates in the orbit and inserts between the tarsal plates of the upper eyelid.
—elevates the upper lid.

Glands of the Lids

—are of three types: meibomian glands, glands of Moll, and the glands of Zeis.

Meibomian Glands

—are elongated sebaceous glands located in the tarsal plates of the eyelids.
—their oily secretion is delivered behind the eyelashes at the free edge of the eyelids and retards rapid evaporation of tears from the eye.

Glands of Zeis

—are modified sebaceous glands associated with hair follicles.

Glands of Moll
—are sweat glands that empty into the eyelash hair follicles.
—infection of these latter two types of glands results in a sty.

Lacrimal Apparatus
—consists of the lacrimal gland, lacrimal canaliculi, lacrimal sac, and the nasolacrimal duct.

Lacrimal Gland
—is a tear gland (compound tubuloalveolar) located in the anterolateral aspect of the orbit.
—its cells contain secretory granules and are surrounded, in part, by an incomplete layer of myoepithelial cells.
—empties its secretions (tears) into the conjunctival fornix via 6 to 12 ducts from which the tears flow over the cornea and conjunctive, keeping them moist.

Tears
—flow to the medial aspect of the eye and enter the lacrimal puncta, which drains into the lacrimal canaliculi.
—contain the enzyme lysozyme, an antibacterial agent.

Lacrimal Canaliculi
—drain the lacrimal puncta, which are openings located in the medial margin of each eyelid.
—are lined with a stratified squamous epithelium, and they unite to form a common canaliculus that empties into the lacrimal sac.

Lacrimal Sac
—is a reservoir of the lacrimal apparatus.
—is located in the nasolacrimal fossa of the orbit.
—receives tears from the lacrimal canaliculus and is lined by a pseudostratified ciliated columnar epithelium.

Nasolacrimal Duct
—is the inferior continuation of the lacrimal sac and is housed in the bony nasolacrimal fossa.
—is lined by a pseudostratified ciliated columnar epithelium and terminates by emptying its contents into the inferior meatus of the nasal cavity.

Ear

Ear (vestibulocochlear apparatus)
—functions in hearing and equilibrium.
—has three regions: external ear, middle ear, and inner ear.

External Ear (pinna)
—receives sound waves, which impinge upon the tympanic membrane (eardrum).

Middle Ear
—is the space housing the three bony ossicles (malleus, incus, and stapes) that transmit the vibrations received by the tympanic membrane.

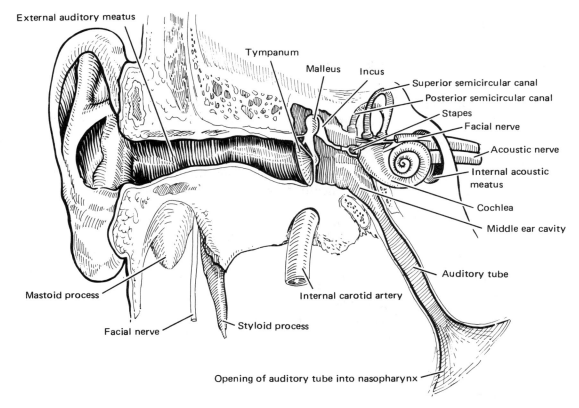

Figure 19.5. Diagram of the external, middle, and internal ears. (From Hiatt JL, Gartner LP: *Textbook of Head and Neck Anatomy*, ed 2. Baltimore, Williams & Wilkins, 1987.)

Stapes

—(last bone in the series) vibrates the membrane covering the oval window of the inner ear.

Inner Ear

—(housed within the bony cochlea) contains cavities and canals filled with fluid (endolymph and perilymph).

—housed here also are the semicircular canals, utricle, and saccule, structures specialized to access and evaluate equilibrium.

—fluid-filled sacs of the membranous labyrinth containing these structures has specialized nerve (hair) cells.

—movement of the fluid within the labyrinth stimulates the hair cells, which triggers an impulse that is transmitted via the vestibular portion of the acoustic nerve to the brain.

—changes in the orientation of the semicircular canals and other portions of the vestibular apparatus permit an evaluation of head movements, their orientation, and changes in their velocity and direction.

Fluid

—set in motion by movements at the oval window stimulates specialized nerve cells that generate nerve impulses that travel via the acoustic nerve to the brain.

External Ear

Auricle (pinna)

—is the external ear composed of irregular plates of elastic cartilage covered by thin skin, containing hair follicles, sebaceous glands, and a few sweat glands.

External Auditory Meatus

—is the skin-lined canal leading to and terminating at the tympanic membrane (where the middle ear begins).

Skin

—is a stratified squamous keratinized epithelium containing hair follicles, sebaceous glands, and ceruminous glands (modified sweat glands), which produce earwax (cerumen).

—deep to the skin, the wall of the external auditory canal is composed of elastic cartilages (in the outer third) and bone (in the inner two-thirds).

Tympanic Membrane

—(eardrum) is the thin membrane covering the deepest aspect of the external auditory meatus.

—its external surface is covered by stratified squamous keratinized epithelium.

—its internal surface is lined by a simple cuboidal epithelium.

—possesses fibroelastic connective tissue interposed between these two epithelial coverings.

Middle Ear

Tympanic Cavity

—is a small irregular space lying between the tympanic membrane and the inner ear (within the temporal bone).

—is lined by a simple squamous epithelium.

—is connected to the pharynx via the auditory tube (eustachian tube).

—also communicates with the air-filled cavities in the mastoid process.

—is lined by a pseudostratified ciliated columnar epithelium.

—its lamina propria, composed of dense connective tissue, is tightly adherent to the bony wall, except in the areas where the oval and round windows are present.

Ossicles

—are arranged in series: the malleus (attached to the tympanic membrane) articulates with the incus, which in turn articulates with the stapes, which is attached to the oval window.

—transmit movements of the tympanic membrane to the oval window.

Reflex Action

—of two small muscles, the tensor tympani attached to the malleus and the stapedius attached to the stapes, prevent the ossicles from damaging the oval window when loud sounds are being transmitted.

Internal Ear

Inner Ear

—is composed of a bony labyrinth located within the temporal bone that houses the membranous labyrinth.

Bony Labyrinth
—is composed of irregular spaces within the temporal bone.
—includes the three semicircular canals with their semicircular ducts, the vestibule and the cochlea.

Vestibule
—is an irregular central area, which houses the utricle and saccule.

Cochlea
—(about 35 mm long) spirals 2.5 times around a bony spiral core, the modiolus, where blood vessels and the spiral ganglion are present.
—contains the cochlear duct.
—osseous spiral lamina is the lateral extension of the modiolus.

Perilymph
—fills the bony labyrinth of the vestibule and the semicircular canals.

Membranous Labyrinth
—is contained within the bony labyrinth.
—is lined by a simple squamous epithelium and contains endolymph.
—has two specialized regions: the maculae-containing utricle and the saccule (sensory structure).
—contains cristae (sensory structures) located in semicircular ducts and spiral organ of Corti.

Saccule and Utricle
—endolymph-filled cavities lined by simple squamous epithelium containing maculae.

Maculae
—are specialized sensory regions located within the epithelium of the saccule and utricle.
—are composed of different epithelial types: two types of neuroepithelial hair cells and supporting cells.
—their free surface is covered by a gelatinous material (probably secreted by the supporting cells) containing small calcified particles, the otoliths.

Gelatinous Layer (otolithic membrane)
—is arranged vertically in the saccule and horizontally in the utricle, so that linear acceleration (positive or negative) of the head in these two planes is detected by the central nervous system.

Hair Cells
—are of two types and distinguished primarily by their type of afferent innervation, although they also vary somewhat in shape.

Type I Neuroepithelial Hair Cells
—are bulbar in shape. The expanded portion contains a round nucleus, numerous mitochondria, and a well-developed Golgi apparatus.
—their free surface displays 50 to 100 elongated rigid sensory microvilli (stereocilia) arranged in rows and a single cilium (kinocilium).
—is almost completely surrounded by a cup-shaped nerve ending, which sometimes contains dense linear structures resembling synaptic ribbons (seen in the retina).

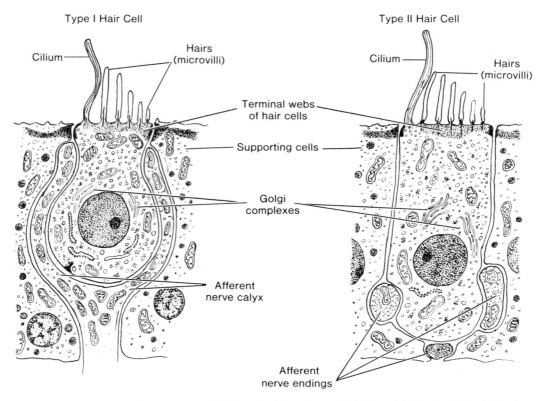

Figure 19.6. Diagrams of type I and type II hair cells. (From Krause WJ, Cutts JH: *Concise Text of Histology*, ed 2. Baltimore, Williams & Wilkins, 1985.)

Type II Neuroepithelial Hair Cells
—are columnar in shape, possess basally located round nuclei, and have many mitochondria and a well-developed Golgi apparatus.
—their free surface displays 50 to 100 long rigid microvilli (stereocilia) arranged in rows and a single cilium (kinocilium).

Small Afferent Terminals
—(containing synaptic vesicles) make contact with these cells, and occasionally "synaptic ribbons" are present in the hair cells near these sites.

Supporting Cells
—occupy the spaces between the hair cells.
—are columnar cells but extremely complex in shape, occluding the space available between the hair cells.
—their nuclei are round and basally located.
—possess many microtubules that project from the base of the cell into an extensive terminal web.

Endolymphatic Duct
—formed by the union of narrow ducts, ends in an expanded endolymphatic sac.

Endolymphatic Sac
—epithelial lining contains two types of columnar cells.

Electron-Dense Cell

—has an irregularly shaped nucleus.

Electron-Lucent Cell

—has long microvilli, many pinocytotic vesicles, and vacuoles.
—may function in resorption of endolymph.

Phagocytic Cells (macrophages, neutrophils)

—cross the epithelium to phagocytose debris and foreign materials in the endolymphatic sac.

Semicircular Ducts

—are located in the semicircular canals.
—are three in number and are oriented perpendicular to each other.
—contain endolymph that communicates with that in the utricle and the saccule.
—each possesses a dilated region, the ampulla, which houses the crista, a sensory structure that resembles a macula.

Cristae

—of the three semicircular ducts are positioned perpendicular to each other; therefore, angular acceleration along any of the three axes is detected.

Crista Ampullaris

—is a sensory receptor site composed of two types of neuroepithelial hair cells and supporting cells. Free surfaces of these cells are covered by a thick glycoprotein layer of material called the cupula.

Cupula

—has a conical shape over the receptor cells, and it contains no otoliths.

Cochlear Duct

—is a specialized diverticulum of the saccule that contains the spiral organ of Corti, which responds to various sound frequencies.
—contains endolymph, is bordered by two perilymph-containing structures, the scala vestibuli (above) and the scala tympani (below).
—scalae communicate with each other at the helicotrema, located at the apex of the cochlea.

Spiral Organ of Corti

—is supported on its medial aspect by a bony outcropping, the modiolus, and its lateral projection is known as the osseous spiral lamina.
—periosteum of the osseous spiral lamina is modified to form the spiral limbus, whose superior surface contains the interdental cells.
—lateral aspect of the spiral organ of Corti, positioned away from the modiolus, is supported by the thickened periosteum of the cochlea, known as the spiral ligament.
—basilar membrane is a thin membrane that extends between the spiral ligament and the osseous spiral lamina.

Vestibular Membrane

—stretches across the cochlear duct and is composed of two layers of flattened squamous epithelial cells, separated from each other by an intervening basal lamina.

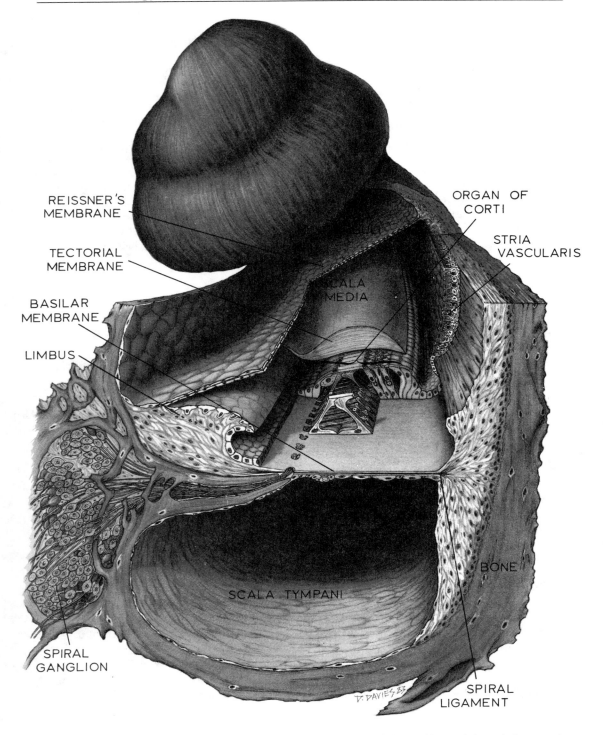

REISSNER'S
MEMBRANE

TECTORIAL
MEMBRANE

BASILAR
MEMBRANE

LIMBUS

SPIRAL
GANGLION

ORGAN OF
CORTI

STRIA
VASCULARIS

SCALA
MEDIA

BONE

SCALA TYMPANI

SPIRAL
LIGAMENT

D. DAVIES 83

Figure 19.7. Schematic diagram illustrating the various components of the cochlea and the spiral organ of Corti. (From Kelly DE, Wood RL, Enders AC: *Bailey's Textbook of Microscopic Anatomy*, ed 18. Baltimore, Williams & Wilkins, 1984.)

Stria Vascularis
—a modified epithelial lining of the lateral aspect of the cochlear duct, consists of a pseudostratified epithelium composed of three types of cells, basal, intermediate, and marginal cells, and is vascularized by capillaries.
—probably secretes endolymph.
—basal cells are electron lucent, contain few mitochondria, and interdigitate with the intermediate cells that closely invest the capillaries located within this epithelium.
—marginal cells are more electron dense and contain many mitochondria and microvilli.

Spiral Prominence
—is a protuberance covered by epithelium that extends the length of the cochlear duct.
—its epithelium is continuous with that of the stria vascularis (above) and is reflected onto the basilar membrane, where it follows an indentation to form the external spiral sulcus.
—its cells become cuboidal and continue onto the basilar membrane, where they are known as the cells of Claudius.

Cells of Claudius
—overlie the polyhedral-shaped cells of Boettcher.
—numerous microvilli extending from the cells of Boettcher suggest that they have secretory and/or absorptive functions.

Spiral Organ of Corti
—responds to different sound frequencies.
—lies upon both parts of the basilar membrane (zona pectinata and zona arcuata).
—is composed of inner and outer hair cells and supporting cells (inner and outer pillar cells, inner and outer phalangeal cells, border cells, and the cells of Hensen).
—displays two tunnels: the inner tunnel of Corti and the outer tunnel (space of Nuell).
—inner tunnel of Corti spans the length of the cochlea and is enclosed by the inner and outer pillar cells.
—outer tunnel (space of Nuel) is located between the cells of Hensen and the outer hair cells.
—tunnels communicate with each other via intercellular spaces.

Inner Hair Cells
—are neuroepithelial.
—function in the reception of sound.
—are organized as a single row of cells along the entire length of the cochlea.
—are bulbous in shape, their nuclei are basally located, and they contain many mitochondria (concentrated around the nucleus).
—their free surface displays many elongated stiff stereocilia arranged in a W-shaped formation and possesses a basal body but lacks a kinocilium.
—basal aspect of the cell receives numerous afferent synaptic terminals.

Outer Hair Cells
—are neuroepithelial and organized in three or more rows located between the outer phalangeal and outer pillar cells.
—are couched in recesses formed by the outer phalangeal cells.

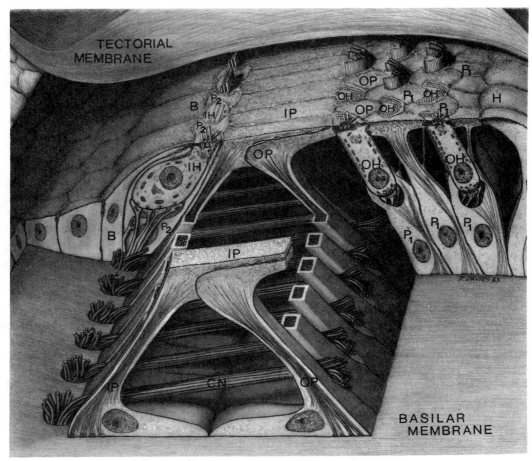

Figure 19.8. Schematic illustration of the spiral organ of Corti. (From Kelly DE, Wood RL, Enders AC: *Bailey's Textbook of Microscopic Anatomy*, ed 18. Baltimore, Williams & Wilkins, 1984.)

—their nuclei are round, basally located, and surrounded by many mitochondria.
—their free surface has many long stiff stereocilia that are arranged in a W formation.
—their basal plasma membrane is ensconced in cup-shaped afferent nerve endings that make synaptic contact with it.
—possess a basal body but no kinocilium.

Inner and Outer Pillar Cells

—are intimately associated with each other, and they both rest on the basilar membrane.
—are supportive cells.
—enclose a space, the inner tunnel of Corti.
—possess a wide base and have elongated processes that contain microtubules, intermediate filaments, and microfilaments (actin).

Inner and Outer Phalangeal Cells

—are the supportive elements that are intimately associated with the inner and outer hair cells, respectively.
—support the slender nerve fibers that form synapses with the hair cells.

Cells of Hensen and Border Cells

—delineate the inner and outer borders of the spiral organ of Corti.
—cells of Hensen are continuous with the cells of Claudius.
—border cells continue into the region of the inner phalangeal cells.

Tectorial Membrane

—is a glycoprotein-rich, viscous material overlying the tips of the hair cells.
—is secreted by the interdental cells of the spiral sulcus.

Basilar Membrane

—is a thick layer of amorphous material that contains keratin-like fibrils.
—extends from the spiral ligament to the tympanic lip of the limbus spiralis.
—is subdivided into two regions: the medial zona arcuata and the lateral zona pectinata.
—is probably manufactured by the mesothelial cells of the scala tympani, although some suggest that cells of the spiral organ of Corti also assist in its formation.
—its vibrations, induced by disturbances in the perilymph, are detected by the hair cells, which transduce the mechanical energy into electrical impulses that travel via the cochlear nerve to the brain.

Oscillations

—set in motion at the oval window are dissipated at the secondary tympanic membrane covering the round window of the cochlea.

REVIEW TESTS

SPECIAL SENSES

DIRECTIONS: *One* or *more* of the given statements or completions is/are correct. Choose answers:

A. if only **1**, **2**, and **3** are correct
B. if only **1** and **3** are correct
C. if only **2** and **4** are correct
D. if only **4** is correct
E. if **all** are correct

19.1. Meissner's corpuscles are found in
1. hairless skin
2. lips
3. nipples
4. serous membranes

19.2. Aqueous humor
1. is produced by the ciliary process
2. flows from the posterior chamber into the anterior chamber
3. exits via the canal of Schlemm
4. is related to glaucoma

19.3. The cornea is
1. the anterior portion of the tunica fibrosa
2. avascular
3. composed of five layers
4. rich in nerve endings

19.4. The choroid
1. is highly vascular
2. is the pigmented layer of the eye
3. is attached to the tunica fibrosa
4. contains no melanocytes

19.5. The membranous labyrinth
1. contains perilymph
2. contains the saccule
3. surrounds the bony labyrinth
4. contains the utricle

DIRECTIONS: Each of the following questions contains four suggested answers. Choose the *one* that is *best* in each case.

19.6. Which of the following is missing in the fovea centralis?
a. rods
b. cones
c. rods and cones
d. choroid

19.7. Communication of the scala vestibuli and scala tympani occurs at the
a. round window
b. oval window
c. helicotrema
d. endolymphatic sac

19.8. The bony ossicles of the middle ear cavity are arranged in a series bridging the tympanic cavity, beginning at the tympanic membrane and ending at the

a. endolymphatic duct
b. round window
c. helicotrema
d. oval window

19.9. Neuroepithelial cells located in the inner ear and connected to the vestibular division of the acoustic nerve are represented by

a. hair cells in the maculae
b. outer pillar cells
c. inner pillar cells
d. cells of Hensen

19.10. Bases of the inner hair cells of the spiral organ of Corti rest upon the

a. tectorial membrane
b. basilar membrane
c. phalangeal cells
d. spiral prominence

DIRECTIONS: The following questions or statements refer to the photomicrographs below (Figures 19.9 and 19.10). The letters on the figures are answers to the numbered items appearing below the photomicrographs. For each numbered item select the *one* letter that *best* corresponds to that item. Each letter may be used once, more than once, or not at all.

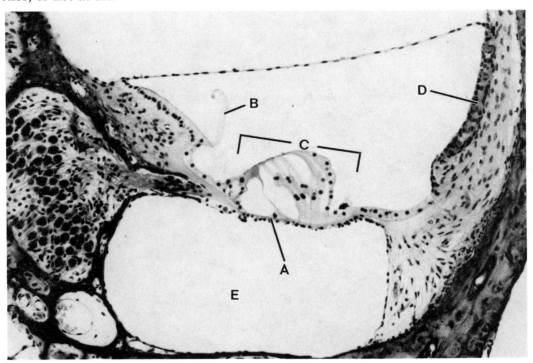

Figure 19.9. From Gartner LP, Hiatt JL: *Atlas of Histology*. Baltimore, Williams & Wilkins, 1987.)

19.11. Spiral organ of Corti

19.12. Basilar membrane

19.13. Scala tympani

19.14. Tectorial membrane

19.15. Stria vascularis

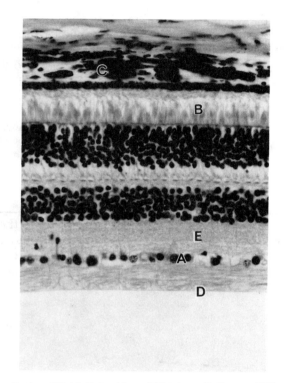

Figure 19.10. From Gartner LP, Hiatt JL: *Atlas of Histology*. Baltimore, Williams & Wilkins, 1987.)

19.16. Choroid

19.17. Layer of rods and cones

19.18. Inner limiting membrane

19.19. Ganglion cell layer

19.20. Inner plexiform layer

ANSWERS AND EXPLANATIONS

SPECIAL SENSES

19.1. A (1, 2, and 3)
Meissner's corpuscles are found in the hairless skin of the lips and the nipples. They are not found in serous membranes.

19.2. E (**all** are correct)
Aqueous humor is produced by the ciliary processes located in the posterior chamber of the eye. From here it flows to the anterior chamber and into the canal of Schlemm. When the canal of Schlemm is blocked a condition called glaucoma exists as the volume of aqueous humor builds and increases the pressure in the eye. If untreated, blindness often results.

19.3. E (**all** are correct)
The cornea is the anterior portion of the tunica fibrosa, the outer covering of the eye. It is composed of five distinct layers and is very rich in sensory nerve endings. It is also avascular.

19.4. A (1, 2, and 3)
The choroid is the vascular, pigmented layer of the eye containing many melanocytes that impart dark pigment to the eye. It is loosely attached to the tunica fibrosa.

19.5. C (2 and 4)
The membranous labyrinth contains the saccule and the utricle and is filled with endolymph. Perilymph is the fluid contained within the bony labyrinth, which lies outside the membranous labyrinth.

19.6. a
The fovea centralis contains the choroid layer and only cones. It represents the area of greatest visual acuity in the retina.

19.7. c
The scala vestibuli and the scala tympani are in reality one perilymphatic space separated by the cochlear duct (scala media). The scalae vestibuli and tympani communicate with each other at the helicotrema.

19.8. d
The bony ossicles of the middle ear cavity articulate in a series from the tympanic membrane to the oval window.

19.9. a
Neuroepithelial hair cells connected to the vestibular portion of the acoustic nerve are found in the maculae of the saccule and the utricle.

19.10. c
The inner neuropithelial hair cells of the spiral organ of Corti are unique in that they do not rest upon the basilar membrane. Instead their bases are supported by the phalangeal cells.

19.11. C, organ of corti

19.12. A, basilar membrane

19.13. E, scala tympani

19.14. B, tectorial membrane

19.15. D, stria vascularis

19.16. C, choroid

19.17. B, layer of rods and cones

19.18. D, inner limiting membrane

19.19. A, ganglion cell layer

19.20. E, inner plexiform layer

INDEX